KETO [

COOKBOOK

AFTER 50

A comprehensive guide to get a better metabolism, burn fat, lose weight prevent diabetes, get a ketogenic body and boost your energy with a tasty meal plan

ALICE HARWING

TABLE OF CONTENTS

Introduction 1

Chapter 01 - What Is A Ketogenic Diet 7

Chapter 02 - What You Can't Eat On A Keto Diet 15

Chapter 03 - Allowed Product List 25

Chapter 04 - The Foods That Can Help To Slow Down Aging.....................35

Chapter 05 - Breakfast...39

Chapter 06 - Appetizers and Side Dishes..61

Chapter 07 - Lunch..77

Chapter 08 - Dinner 101

Chapter 09 - Dessert 131

Chapter 10 - Soup...163

Chapter 11 - Vegetables...185

Chapter 12 - Conclusion 199

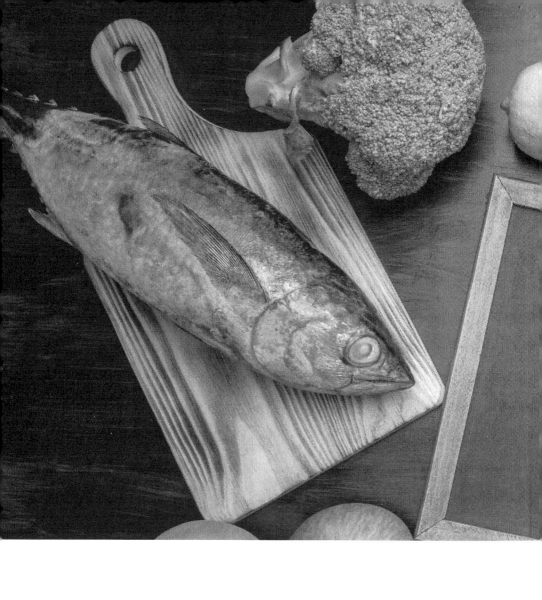

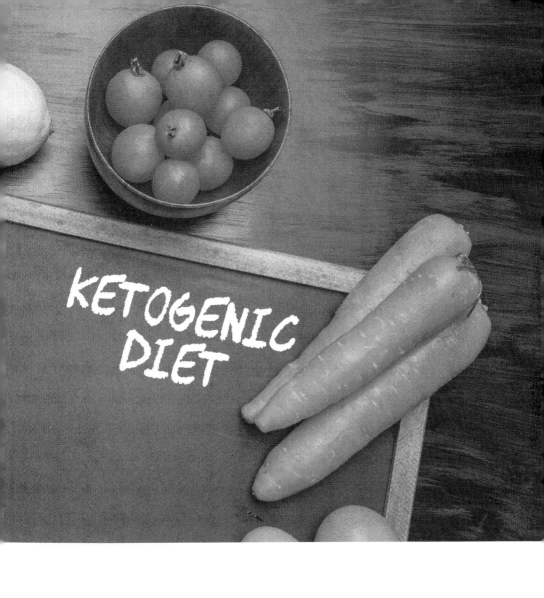

INTRODUCTION

Introduction

When you start at about 50, you will notice a lot of changes in your body, it is more than normal. Among the most common symptoms, there is a loss of muscle, insomnia, finer skin. You don't have to worry about this, but you have to pay much more attention than usual to your lifestyle, it is essential, to keep fit, that you start attending a gym, as well as a healthy and correct diet under all macros.

You can apply it even if you have health problems. Of course, a visit to a nutritionist can help you personalize your diet even more effectively. But this is "something more," the information in this guidebook is more than enough, you just need to study it and apply it diligently.

As said, the functions of our body change according to age, in particular, the thing that changes most is our metabolism, it is physiological that it slows down with age. This change is due both to aging, but also to our lifestyle. Current metabolism is a consequence of our lifestyle in recent years.

A healthy lifestyle, with frequent low-abundance meals, with moderate alcohol consumption, will certainly have a faster metabolism than a lifestyle consisting of large meals eaten once a day, alcohol, and insomnia.

The ketogenic diet can definitely help you from this point of view, eliminating carbohydrates and promoting the elimination of fats from our body. Another advantage is its flexibility, in fact, you can play with macros and adapt them to your needs and your lifestyle, in addition to the progress made, of course.

Start gradually, your body has adapted for years to an unhealthy lifestyle, so do not overdo it overnight. Take your time and slowly reach your goals. There is no need to run, this is a marathon, not 100 meters.

At first, you may feel tired, tired, without energy. Don't worry, it's a normal thing, it's your body that is adapting to the new food style. You're taking away its main source of energy, carbohydrates, it's logical that it has to adapt. It must change the main energy source, it must switch to using fats, but this takes time, two or three days are necessary. The drop in sugars could decrease your pressure for a couple of days, avoid exercise and there will be no problems. The resulting benefits will be enormous.

Consult a nutrition specialist. This guidebook is a very valuable tool to get an idea of what a ketogenic diet is, what the benefits are, how to avoid classic mistakes. It is a complete guide, with which, if studied well, you will certainly be able to set your diet according to your daily needs. However, consulting a doctor is never a bad idea, you can discuss your opinions and can give you valuable advice. I recommend consulting your doctor, especially in cases of health problems and in cases where you have never been on a diet.

This book is filled with delicious keto meals that you can cook in your own home. The recipes in this book are easy to do and complete with preparation time, cooking time, ingredients, directions, and nutritional facts. Read on and let's get started.

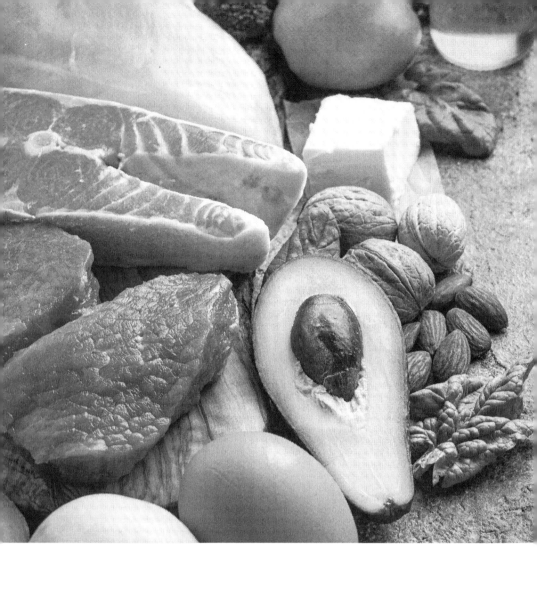

CHAPTER 01

WHAT IS A KETOGENIC DIET

Chapter 01 - What Is A Ketogenic Diet

You are going to receive a glimpse into what the keto weight-reduction plan sincerely is and how it stacks up relative to the other famous diets obtainable on the market. This sort of comparative evaluation would be capable of doing things. One, it will let you gather perspective on the weight loss plan enterprise and the variety of alternatives that might have a purpose worth trying. And, it will offer you a more informed opinion and a more strong resolve for whatever healthy diet weight-reduction plan you do eventually pick to adopt for yourself inside the future.

KETO AS THE BEST DIET PLAN OUT THERE

It's proper that there are undoubtedly many weight loss plan plans obtainable at the market, and it'd be too arrogant to say that the keto weight loss plan is high-quality among them all. However, it would be fair to mention that the keto eating regimen is a high-quality one for you for my part if it takes place to serve your wishes and your goals higher effectively.

The keto food plan is a low-carb diet that is designed to place the human frame into a heightened ketogenic state, which might inevitably result in higher pronounced fat burn and weight loss. It is a reasonably accessible food regimen with a variety of keto-friendly meals being readily available in marketplaces at highly low prices. It isn't an eating regimen that is reserved most effectively for the affluent and elite.

As some distance as effectiveness is concerned, there's just no denying how impactful a keto eating regimen might be for someone who wants to lose a drastic quantity of weight in a wholesome and managed manner. The keto weight-reduction plan also enforces discipline and precision for the agent by incorporating macro counting and meal journaling to ensure accuracy and accountability in the weight-reduction project. There are no external factors that can impact how robust this weight loss plan may be for you. Everything is all within your control.

And lastly, it's a reasonably sustainable weight loss plan, for the reason that it doesn't merely compromise on taste or range. Sure, there are lots of restrictions. But ultimately, there are lots of alternatives and workarounds that can assist stave off cravings. If these kinds of standards and reasons observe to you and your personal life, then it could genuinely be safe to say that the keto food plan is a high-quality one for you.

WHAT SETS KETO APART FROM OTHERS?

But how precisely does keto stack up against other weight loss plan plans obtainable? Well, if your purpose for dieting is weight loss, then it would be prudent to investigate different diets that are similar to the keto eating regimen's goals of inducing weight reduction and fats burn. You should advantage a higher understanding of these diets and why the keto eating regimen would, in all likelihood, nonetheless be the better one for you. The three foods which are most usually compared to the keto weight loss plan in phrases of meal composition and bodily effects are Atkins, paleo, and Whole30.

ATKINS

The Atkins and keto diets are so similar in the feel that they both promote a high intake of fat, mild consumption of protein, and minimum intake of carbohydrates. Typically, while on Atkins, a person's typical diet would be composed of 60% fat, 30% protein, and 10% carbohydrates. This is still a relatively minimal carbohydrate composition even when you take into consideration the keto breakdown of 75% fat, 20% protein, and 5% carbohydrates.

The problem with Atkins isn't found in better carbohydrate consumption. It's, in most cases, located inside the elevated consumption of protein. Any extra protein that the body doesn't dissipate for muscle constructing or repair is converted into glucose. And that glucose goes to be used for energy in preference to the stored fat that you could have, at this moment making the metabolic fee of your frame slower. The keto diet nonetheless offers you the protein blessings of constructing and repairing muscles without compromising the advantages of ketosis at the same time.

PALEO

The paleo food regimen is one that is gaining full-size popularity in the cutting-edge health industry. It stems from the studied nutritional practices of the Paleolithic era, which was depending on the hunter-gatherer system of food rationing and production. It is a food regimen that focuses entirely on complete ingredients that are free from any processing. Food items which include wheat, grains, dairy, legumes, processed sugars, processed oils, corn, processed fats, etc. are prohibited. It specializes in the high intake of meats and non-starchy greens.

Like the keto weight-reduction plan, the paleo diet additionally takes place to be a low-carb diet that emphasizes a better consumption of fat and proteins. However, it doesn't indeed restrict the wide variety of carbohydrates or energy that a person might take on day by day basis. It's a weight loss plan that focuses entirely on the composition of meals without the quantity of it, and that may be problematic for several people who've very particular bodily composition dreams.

WHOLE30

Whole30 is a stricter model of the paleo weight-reduction plan. It is a diet plan that is primarily dependent on a thirty-day application of strict eating under paleo principles. It removes the consumption of processed foods, starchy vegetables and carbohydrates, sweeteners, dairy products, legumes, and higher. Once the thirty-day period is over, you're then recommended to reintroduce certain food groups step by step in your weight-reduction plan and examine what kind of impact or effect these will have on you. This is how you will be capable of discovering what type of food you've got a trendy intolerance to.

However, the Whole30 weight loss program doesn't certainly issue in macro counting and calorie counting either. That manner that humans at the Whole30 weight loss plan are nevertheless at risk of gaining weight and getting fat despite the restrictive nature of the weight loss program.

Chapter 02 - What You Can't Eat On A Keto Diet

will show you the kinds of food you want to avoid at all costs. Because keto is a keto diet, that means you need to avoid high-carbs food. Some of the food you avoid is even healthy, but they just contain too many carbs. Here is a list of common food you should limit or avoid altogether.

BREAD AND GRAINS

Bread is a staple food in many countries. You have loaves, bagels, tortillas, and the list goes on. However, no matter what form bread takes, they still pack many carbs. The same applies to whole-grain as well because they are made from refined flour.

Depending on your daily carb limit, eating a sandwich or bagel can put you way over your daily limit. So if you want to eat bread, it is best to make keto variants at home instead.

Grains such as rice, wheat, and oats pack many carbs as well. So limit or avoid that as well.

FRUITS

Fruits are healthy for you. They have been linked to a lower risk of heart disease and cancer. However, there are a few that you need to avoid in your keto diets. The problem is that some of those foods pack quite a lot of carbs such as banana, raisins, dates, mango, and pear.

As a general rule, avoid sweet and dried fruits. Berries are an exception because they do not contain as much sugar and are rich in fiber. So you can still eat some of them, around 50 grams. Moderation is key.

VEGETABLES

Vegetables are just as healthy for your body. Most of the keto diet does not care how many vegetables you eat so long as they are low in starch. Vegetables that are rich in fiber can help with weight loss. For one, they make you feel full for longer, so they help suppress your appetite. Another benefit is that your body would burn more calories to break and digest them. Moreover, they help control blood sugar and aid with your bowel movements.

But that also means you need to avoid or limit vegetables that are high in starch because they have more carbs than fiber. That includes corn, potato, sweet potato, and beets.

PASTA

Pasta is also a staple food in many countries. It is versatile and convenient. As with any other convenient food, pasta is rich in carbs. So when you are on your keto diet, spaghetti or any other types of pasta are not recommended. You can probably get away with it by eating a small portion, but that is not possible.

Thankfully, that does not mean you need to give up on it altogether. If you are craving pasta, you can try some other alternatives that are low in carbs such as spiralized veggies or shirataki noodles.

CEREAL

Cereal is also a huge offender because sugary breakfast cereals pack many carbs. That also applies to "healthy cereals." Just because they use other words to describe their product does not mean that you should believe them. That also applies to oatmeal, whole-grain cereals, etc.

So when you eat a bowl of cereal when you are doing keto, you are already way over your carb limit, and we haven't even added milk into the equation! Therefore, avoid whole-grain cereal or cereals that we mention here altogether.

BEER

In reality, you can drink most alcoholic beverages in moderation without fear. For instance, dry wine does not have that many carbs, and hard liquor has no carbs at all. So you can drink them without worry. Beer is an exception to this rule because it packs a lot of carbs.

Carbs in beers or other liquid are considered to be liquid carbs, and they are even more dangerous than solid carbs. You see, when you eat food that is rich in carbs, you at least feel full. When you drink liquid carbs, you do not feel full as quickly, so the appetite suppression effect is little.

Sweetened Yogurt

Yogurt is very healthy because it is tasty and does not have that many carbs. It is a very versatile food to have in your keto diet. The problem comes when you consume yogurt variants that are rich in carbs such as fruit-flavored, low-fat, sweetened, or nonfat yogurt. A single serving of sweetened yogurt contains as many carbs as a single serving of dessert.

If you love yogurt, you can get away with half a cup of plain Greek yogurt with 50 grams of raspberries or blackberries.

Juice

Fruit juices are perhaps the worst beverage you can put into your system when you are on a keto diet. One may argue that juice provides some nutrients, but the problem is that it contains many carbs that are very easy to digest. As a result, your blood sugar level will spike whenever you drink it. That also applies to vegetable juice because of the fast-digesting carbs present.

Another problem is that the brain does not process liquid carbs the same way as solid carbs. Solid carbs can help suppress appetite, but liquid carbs will only put your appetite into overdrive.

Low-Fat and Fat-Free Salad Dressings

Fruits and vegetables are largely okay, so long as they are low in carbs. But if you have to buy salads, keep in mind that commercial dressings pack more carbs than you think, especially the fat-free and low-fat variants.

So if you want to enjoy your salad, dress your salad using creamy, full-fat dressing instead. To cut down on carbs, you can use vinegar and olive oil, both of which are proven to help with heart health and aid in weight loss.

BEANS AND LEGUMES

These are also very nutritious as they are rich in fiber. Research has shown that eating these have many health benefits, such as reduced inflammation and heart disease risk.

However, they are also rich in carbs. You may be able to enjoy a small amount of them when you are on your keto diet, but make sure you know exactly how much you can eat before you exceed your carb limit.

SUGAR

We mean sugar in any form, including honey. You may already be aware of what foods that contain lots of sugar, such as cookies, candies, and cake, are forbidden on a keto diet or any other form of diet that is designed to lose weight.

What you may not be aware of is that nature's sugar, such as honey, is just as rich in carbs as processed sugar. Natural forms of sugar contain even more carbs.

Not only that sugar, in general, is rich in carbs, they also add little to no nutritional value to your meal. When you are on a keto diet, you need to keep in mind that your diet is going to consist of food that is rich in fiber and nutritious. So sugar is out of the question.

If you want to sweeten your food, you can just use a healthy sweetener instead because they do not add as many carbs to your food.

CHIPS AND CRACKERS

These two are some of the most popular snacks. What some people did not realize is that one packet of chips contain several servings and should not be all eaten in one go. The carbs can add up very quickly if you do not watch what you eat.

Crackers also pack many carbs, although the amount varies based on how they are made. But even whole-wheat crackers contain many carbs.

Due to how processed snacks are produced, it is difficult to stop yourself from eating everything within a short period. Therefore, it is advised that you avoid them altogether.

MILK

Cereal contains many carbs, and a breakfast cereal will put you way over your carbs limit without you adding milk. Milk also contains many carbs on its own. Therefore, avoid it if you can even though milk is a good source of many nutrients such as calcium, potassium, and other B vitamins.

Of course, that does not mean that you have to ditch milk altogether. You can get away with a tablespoon or two of milk for your coffee. But cream or half-and-half is better if you drink coffee frequently. These two contain very few carbs. But if you love to drink milk in large amounts or need it to make your favorite drinks, consider using coconut milk or unsweetened almond instead.

GLUTEN-FREE BAKED GOODS

Wheat, barley, and rye all contain gluten. Some people who have celiac disease still want to enjoy these delicacies but unable to because their gut will become inflamed in response to gluten. As such, gluten-free variants have been created to cater to their needs.

Gluten-free diets are very popular nowadays, but what many people don't seem to realize is that they pack quite a lot of carbs. That includes gluten-free bread, muffins, and other baked products. In reality, they contain even more carbs than their glutenous variant. Moreover, the flour used to make these gluten-free products are made from grains and starches. So when you consume a gluten-free bread, your blood sugar level spikes.

So, just stick to whole foods. Alternatively, you can use almond or coconut flour to make your low-carb bread.

Chapter 03 - Allowed Product List

FATS

Your daily consumption of fats will be around 70% of your food intake. This needs to be high-quality fat that stays in your system to be used as energy. These are typically found in fats that are the result of raw foods and animals.

Some of the best fats for keto are:

- Hard Cheeses
- Nuts like almonds, walnuts, pecans, and macadamia
- Seeds from sunflowers, pumpkins, chia, flaxseed and hemp hearts
- Natural oils like olive oil and coconut oil
- The cacao of at least 85% cacao. This must be unsweetened and unprocessed chocolate
- Poultry, especially dark meat
- Fatty fish
- Whole eggs, especially the yolks
- Whole milk produces like whole milk mozzarella and ricotta
- Cheese

When we look at high-fat foods, cheese tops the list. It is high in fat and has no carbohydrates. Unfortunately, cheese contains many calories, along with unhealthy saturated fats. When you are consuming cheese, be mindful of the amount you eat. Some cheese is a healthy snack and a good alternative to chips and sugary snack items. Small amounts of cheese in your diet, a few ounces daily, will help you control your hunger because it is filling. It has also been found that calcium in cheese may have a positive effect on blood pressure and cholesterol. Consumption of cheese has also been found to increase muscle mass.

NUTS

As you choose which nuts you're going to eat on keto, be sure to take note of the net carbs. Some nuts have more fat than others, and some have more calories and carbohydrates than others. Choose nuts that will fit well in your macros. Because of the high calories and carbs eat nuts in moderation. They may also have a significant amount of protein when eating a large quantity. Be sure you are adhering to your protein macros as well as your carbohydrate macros.

SEEDS

The good thing about seeds about keto is that the carbohydrates are mostly offset by fiber. That makes the net carbohydrates friendly for keto. Seeds tend to be high in fat and contain some protein. However, they often contain harmful omega-6 fatty acids. You can benefit from the normal concentration of nutrients in seeds, but eating them sprouted. To sprout seeds, simply germinate the seeds between two wet paper towels and leave them to sit for 2 to 8 days. Make sure your paper towel remains moist. Eventually, the stem will sprout from the seed. It's still high in nutrients but easier to digest.

OILS

Oils can be your best cooking aid in the keto diet. They must be able to burn at high temperatures to be most effective for cooking. It is important to use unsaturated fats to provide the most heart-healthy oils. The polyunsaturated oils will be a good addition to the fats consumed on a keto like nut oils and avocado oils. These will assist you in achieving a healthy, effective keto diet. Avocado oil, sesame oil, coconut oil, and olive oil have essential qualities to aid in digestion and nutrient absorption. Also, coconut oil speeds up metabolism.

MEAT/FISH/EGGS/DAIRY

Unprocessed meats do not contain carbohydrates, and many are high in fat. Grass-fed meats are better than grain-fed but watch the portion size. Be careful not to exceed the protein requirements in your daily macros. Fish is good, especially fish high in fat like salmon. Avoid the breading, which has carbohydrates. Again, wild-caught fish is better. It is fed naturally off of foods fish are accustomed to eating. This reduces the chance that growth hormones and antibiotics may be included in the feed from farm fat raised fish. Along the same lines, try to stick to cage-free pasture-raised eggs in the hopes of avoiding chemical additives that might reduce the quality of the food you are consuming. The same is true for milk. Milk and dairy products should be organic to avoid growth hormones and antibiotics that may be found in conventional Foods today. Meat fish eggs and dairy are high in fat; I can be a good source of the fat you need to consume on the keto diet.

PROTEINS

Protein will make up 20% of your daily food intake. It is important not to exceed your protein macros. Be sure you're making good decisions regarding your protein if a person that you are including your diet. It will be consuming a lot of fat, which may contain much protein. So you have to be sure to combine your fat macros with your protein macros when you're setting up your meal plan for the day.

Some of the proteins that you will be eating that are most efficient are:

- Salmon
- Mackerel
- Tuna
- Sardines
- Eggs
- Greek yogurt

- Shrimp
- Chicken thighs
- Peanuts
- Pistachios
- Almonds
- Soybeans (edamame)

NUT BUTTER

The goal of the keto diet is not to eat low-fat proteins. Luckily, there are many high-fat proteins available for consumption. Many times, you will be able to satisfy your fat macros and protein macros with the same food items. Watch your calories, and be sure to incorporate your snack foods into your protein count. Be mindful that green leafy vegetables also contain protein.

It is important to consume enough protein so that carbohydrates in your body do not use muscle to convert to energy. Conversely, too much protein can cause muscle tissue to break down and turn into sugar because of the lack of carbohydrates available on a low-carb diet. Eat the right amount of protein, and don't forget about adding in the protein found snacks and vegetables, especially cream hidden ones when considering your protein macros.

FISH

Some of the best foods for protein on keto are fatty proteins found in salmon, mackerel, and sardines. These proteins are high in fat and omega-3 fatty acids. Fresh fish is higher in omega-3 fatty acid than canned fish, but if you are going to eat fish protein, make sure it is high in fat. This is an efficient way to consume protein and fat that will be converted to energy.

EGGS

Some studies indicate that people who include dairy in their diet have less hunger, and the consumption of dairy may inhibit the production of cortisol, and therefore, the resulting abdominal fat. Full-fat dairy is high in calories, so be sure not to over-consume. It is common for conventional milk and dairy products to contain growth hormones. Dairy from grass-fed animals and organic dairy products are recommended. Aside from the hormones, conventional dairy products do not have as high levels of omega-3 fatty acids, which have anti-inflammatory qualities and promote joint health. Dairy contains much protein. If you're eating meat protein, you should be especially cognizant of the amount of dairy that you're eating so you do not exceed your protein macros. Egg whites are lower in calories and contain the protein of the egg. The egg yolks contain the fat of eggs. If you're going to eat meat and eggs and you have consumed enough fat for the daily macro, you may be able to eat the white instead of the yolks without adding additional fat. The yolk also carries the bulk of calories from eggs, and egg whites have very few calories.

NUTS/NUT BUTTERS/SOYBEANS

Nuts and soybeans (edamame) make excellent snack foods on keto. Eating good quality protein and protein-filled snacks, especially after exercising, may assist your body in building muscle. Snacks should be kept small. They should simply be a means to curb your hunger pains. That is why a quick snack of nuts is ideal. They contain some proteins, some fats, and some carbohydrates. Count the nuts you select to be sure you don't eat too many carbs. Carefully measure the serving size of your snack. Since nuts are small, it is easy to think that eating a few extra nuts here and there won't matter. Whether this is true depends on the nut. That's a good way to add moderate levels of protein to your diet and to adjust your protein macros for the day.

CARBOHYDRATES

So far, it has been stressed to eat more fat, the correct amount of protein, and now, it is time for carbohydrates. Eat fewer carbohydrates. Consume 10% of your daily food in the form of carbohydrates. This is the crux of the ketogenic diet. Normally, carbohydrates are limited to 5% of the daily calories eaten. In doing the gentle keto, the carbohydrates are increased to 10%. Whether 5% or 10%, be sure to minimize the number of carbohydrates in your diet. Also, try to make the carbohydrates of good quality that will burn off quickly so that your body moves quickly to burning fat.

There are many no-carb options available when eating fats and protein. What is needed to add to your diet are vegetables. Produce has nutrients and vitamins that your body needs, so they should be included in your diet. Be sure to incorporate foods that have valuable nutrients such as vegetables and berries into your diet. These are low in carbohydrates. Some of the vegetables and fruits should be used more sparingly than others. Look at green leafy vegetables and vegetables that grow above the ground as low carbohydrate options to provide healthy options that will not add fat. Vegetables that grow underground like carrots and potatoes tend to have more sugar content and are higher in carbohydrates.

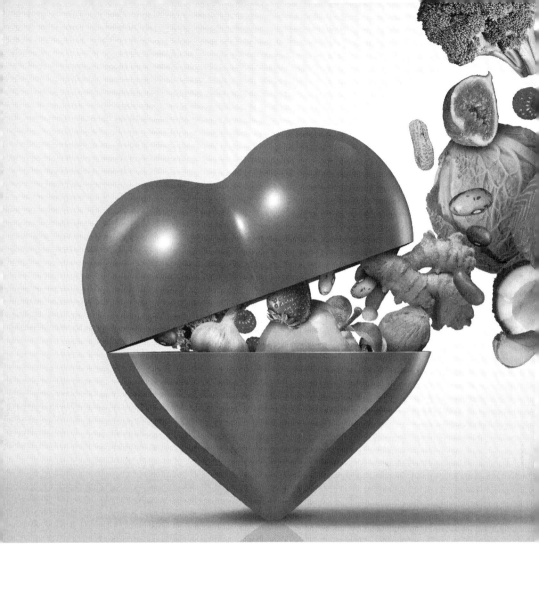

CHAPTER
04

THE FOODS THAT CAN HELP
TO SLOW DOWN AGING

Chapter 04 - The Foods That Can Help To Slow Down Aging

our food intake for the day should be as clean as possible because this can help you to get a youthful look. Consider looking into whole foods diets such as Paleo, Juicing, or Plant-Strong, since these are simple to follow and will give you the basics of how to cut out processed and toxin-filled junk. Most of these diets are not expensive despite what you may think and you might actually find yourself saving money as well as losing weight. Whole foods are good because they're often much more filling than junk and because they're rich in all the anti-aging nutrients you could possibly need. In fact, if you're using a food tracker, simply eating cleaner may mean you won't even need a multivitamin or some anti-aging supplements (like high-dose Vitamin C). If at all possible, get your nutrients from your food, they're better quality and much easier for the body to absorb than the pharmaceutical versions. Remember that calorie restriction is important when it comes to eating well for anti-aging.

At the end of your day, head home to another nutritious meal, but don't forget to spend time with people that you care about. Being present in your life will make it much more meaningful, what's the point in living 100 years if you don't enjoy it? By being social and present, you'll also get the anti-aging benefits of doing so as well as create better memories for yourself. Consider getting together to do something active as you'll need to be up and moving at least 30 minutes a day. If you haven't yet done your yoga consider looking into partner-yoga or classes together. Partner yoga is an ideal way to bring you closer together too. If possible, try to do this in places of nature. Being around nature has been proven to have a positive impact on the brain.

If you're going to head to the gym, try and find one that has a sauna. The reason for this is that sweating is one of the most efficient ways for your body to get rid of toxins. Cigarette smoke and sun damage can all age your skin through toxins, but these are quickly sweated out in a sauna. Studies have shown that by using a sauna regularly, you can help reduce the appearance of wrinkles temporarily. As the steam penetrates the skin, the pores open up, releasing anything in the cells to the steam. You'll only need to spend 10-20 minutes in there to feel the beneficial effects.

Don't forget your supplement regime throughout the day. Many anti-aging supplements need to be taken at specific times or with meals, so plan your supplements accordingly and consider getting a pill organizer if you can't remember them.

When you finally head to bed, you'll want to make sure that you're moisturizing your skin again. If you didn't make your 8 glasses of water, consider having one before bed to top up what you've missed. A hot cup of tea is also an ideal way to relax before bed. Lavender oil has many anti-aging properties and is also great for relaxation. You can take lavender as a relaxing tea before bed or put a few drops of the oil onto your pillow before going to bed.

The key to being successful in this plan is that you need to be able to fit as many of these things into your daily routine as possible. It's fairly established that if you can do something for 7 days, then it will become a hàbit, so simply trying to do it for that long before saying you can't is important. But, above all, if you didn't make your 8 glasses, haven't done your yoga, or ate that hamburger – Don't stress about it! A little slip now and then happens, so let it go and remember that tomorrow is another day.

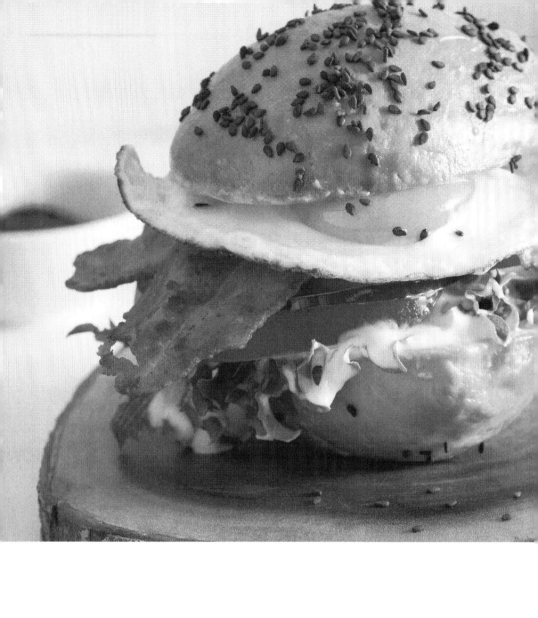

CHAPTER 05

BREAKFAST

BACON CHEESEBURGER WAFFLES

PREPARATION
10 MINS

COOKING
20 MINS

4 SERVINGS

INGREDIENTS

- Toppings

- Pepper and Salt to taste

- 1.5 ounces of cheddar cheese

- 4 tablespoons of sugar-free barbecue sauce

- 4 slices of bacon

- 4 ounces of ground beef, 70% lean meat and 30% fat

- Waffle dough

- Pepper and salt to taste

- 3 tablespoons of parmesan cheese, grated

- 4 tablespoons of almond flour

- ¼ teaspoon of onion powder

- ¼ teaspoon of garlic powder

- 1 cup (125 g) of cauliflower crumbles

- 2 large eggs

- 1.5 ounces of cheddar cheese

NUTRIRION

- Fats: 12g

- Calories: 152g

- Proteins: 6g

- Carbohydrates: 3g

DIRECTIONS

1. Preheat oven to around 350 degrees F.

2. Pulse almonds in a food processor then add in butter and sweetener.

3. Pulse until all the ingredients mix well and coarse dough forms.

4. Coat twelve silicone muffin pans using foil or paper liners.

5. Divide the batter evenly between the muffin pans then press into the bottom part until it forms a crust and bakes for about 8 minutes.

6. In the meantime, mix in a food processor the cream cheese and cottage cheese then pulse until the mixture is smooth.

7. Put in the extracts and sweetener then combine until well mixed.

8. Add in eggs and pulse again until it becomes smooth; you might need to scrape down the mixture from the sides of the processor. Share equally the batter between the muffin pans, then bake for around 30-40 minutes until the middle is not wobbly when you shake the muffin pan lightly.

9. Put aside until cooled completely, then put in the refrigerator for about 2 hours and then top with frozen and thawed berries.

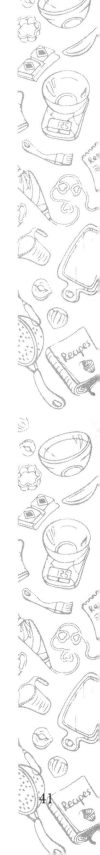

KETO BREAKFAST CHEESECAKE

PREPARATION
20 MINS

COOKING
45 MINS

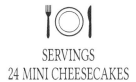

SERVINGS
24 MINI CHEESECAKES

INGREDIENTS

- Toppings

- 1/4 cup of mixed berries for each cheesecake, frozen and thawed

- Filling ingredients

- 1/2 teaspoon of vanilla extract

- 1/2 teaspoon of almond extract

- 3/4 cup of sweetener

- 6 eggs

- 8 ounces of cream cheese

- 16 ounces of cottage cheese

- Crust ingredients

- 4 tablespoons of salted butter

- 2 tablespoons of sweetener

- 2 cups of almonds, whole

NUTRIRION

- Fats: 12g

- Calories: 152g

- Proteins: 6g

- Carbohydrates: 3g

DIRECTIONS

1. Preheat oven to around 350 degrees F.

2. Pulse almonds in a food processor then add in butter and sweetener.

3. Pulse until all the ingredients mix well and coarse dough forms.

4. Coat twelve silicone muffin pans using foil or paper liners.

5. Divide the batter evenly between the muffin pans then press into the bottom part until it forms a crust and bakes for about 8 minutes.

6. In the meantime, mix in a food processor the cream cheese and cottage cheese then pulse until the mixture is smooth.

7. Put in the extracts and sweetener then combine until well mixed.

8. Add in eggs and pulse again until it becomes smooth; you might need to scrape down the mixture from the sides of the processor. Share equally the batter between the muffin pans, then bake for around 30-40 minutes until the middle is not wobbly when you shake the muffin pan lightly.

9. Put aside until cooled completely, then put in the refrigerator for about 2 hours and then top with frozen and thawed berries.

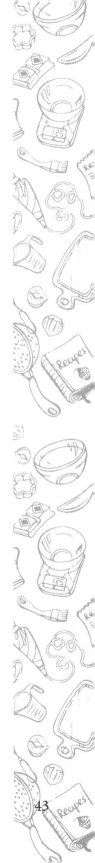

Egg-Crust Pizza

PREPARATION
5 MINS

COOKING
15 MINS

1-2 SERVINGS

INGREDIENTS

- ¼ teaspoon of dried oregano to taste

- ½ teaspoon of spike seasoning to taste

- 1 ounce of mozzarella, chopped into small cubes

- 6 – 8 sliced thinly black olives

- 6 slices of turkey pepperoni, sliced into half

- 4-5 thinly sliced small grape tomatoes

- 2 eggs, beaten well

- 1-2 teaspoons of olive oil

-

NUTRIRION

- Calories: 363g

- Fats: 24.1g

- Carbohydrates: 20.8g

- Proteins: 19.25g

DIRECTIONS

1. Preheat the broiler in an oven than in a small bowl, beat well the eggs. Cut the pepperoni and tomatoes in slices then cut the mozzarella cheese into cubes.

2. Put some olive oil in a skillet over medium heat, then heat the pan for around one minute until it begins to get hot. Add in eggs and season with oregano and spike seasoning, then cook for around 2 minutes until the eggs begin to set at the bottom.

3. Drizzle half of the mozzarella, olives, pepperoni, and tomatoes on the eggs followed by another layer of the remaining half of the above ingredients. Ensure that there is a lot of cheese on the topmost layers. Cover the skillet using a lid and cook until the cheese begins to melt and the eggs are set, for around 3-4 minutes.

4. Place the pan under the preheated broiler and cook until the top has browned and the cheese has melted nicely for around 2-3 minutes. Serve immediately.

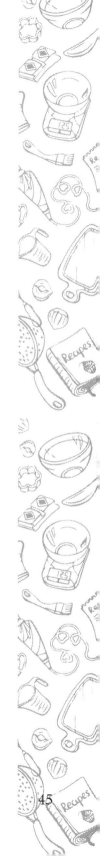

BREAKFAST ROLL-UPS

PREPARATION
5 MINS

COOKING
15 MINS

SERVINGS
5 ROLL-UPS

INGREDIENTS

- Non-stick cooking spray

- 5 patties of cooked breakfast sausage

- 5 slices of cooked bacon

- 1.5 cups of cheddar cheese, shredded

- Pepper and salt

- 10 large eggs

-

NUTRIRION

- Calories: 412.2g

- Fats: 31.66g

- Carbohydrates: 2.26g

- Proteins: 28.21g

DIRECTIONS

1. Preheat a skillet on medium to high heat, then using a whisk, combine two of the eggs in a mixing bowl.

2. After the pan has become hot, lower the heat to medium-low heat then put in the eggs. If you want to, you can utilize some cooking spray.

3. Season eggs with some pepper and salt.

4. Cover the eggs and leave them to cook for a couple of minutes or until the eggs are almost cooked.

5. Drizzle around 1/3 cup of cheese on top of the eggs, then place a strip of bacon and divide the sausage into two and place on top.

6. Roll the egg carefully on top of the fillings. The roll-up will almost look like a taquito. If you have a hard time folding over the egg, use a spatula to keep the egg intact until the egg has molded into a roll-up.

7. Put aside the roll-up then repeat the above steps until you have four more roll-ups; you should have 5 roll-ups in total.

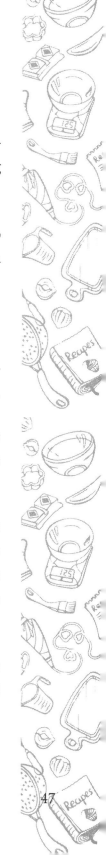

Basic Opie Rolls

PREPARATION
20 MINS

COOKING
35 MINS

SERVINGS
12 ROLLS

INGREDIENTS

- 1/8 teaspoon of salt

- 1/8 teaspoon of cream of tartar

- 3 ounces of cream cheese

- 3 large eggs

NUTRIRION

- Calories: 45

- Fats: 4g

- Carbohydrates: 0g

- Proteins: 2g

DIRECTIONS

1. Preheat the oven to about 300 degrees F, then separate the egg whites from egg yolks and place both eggs in different bowls. Using an electric mixer, beat well the egg whites until the mixture is very bubbly, then add in the cream of tartar and mix again until it forms a stiff peak.

2. In the bowl with the egg yolks, put in 3 ounces of cubed cheese and salt. Mix well until the mixture has doubled in size and is pale yellow. Put in the egg white mixture into the egg yolk mixture then fold the mixture gently together.

3. Spray some oil on the cookie sheet coated with some parchment paper, then add dollops of the batter and bake for around 30 minutes.

4. You will know they are ready when the upper part of the rolls is firm and golden. Leave them to cool for a few minutes on a wire rack. Enjoy with some coffee

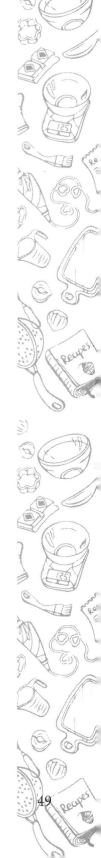

ALMOND COCONUT EGG WRAPS

PREPARATION
5 MINS

COOKING
5 MINS

4 SERVINGS

INGREDIENTS

- 5 Organic eggs

- 1 tbsp Coconut flour

- 25 tsp Sea salt

- 2 tbsp almond meal

NUTRIRION

- Carbohydrates: 3 grams

- Protein: 8 grams

- Fats: 8 grams

- Calories: 111

DIRECTIONS

1. Combine the fixings in a blender and work them until creamy. Heat a skillet using the med-high temperature setting.

2. Pour two tablespoons of batter into the skillet and cook - covered about three minutes. Turn it over to cook for another 3 minutes. Serve the wraps piping hot

Bacon & Avocado Omelet

PREPARATION
5 MINS

COOKING
5 MINS

1 SERVINGS

INGREDIENTS

- 1 slice Crispy bacon

- 2 Large organic eggs

- 5 cup freshly grated parmesan cheese

- 2 tbsp Ghee or coconut oil or butter

- half of 1 small Avocado

NUTRIRION

- Carbohydrates: 3.3 grams

- Protein: 30 grams

- Fats: 63 grams

- Calories: 719

DIRECTIONS

1. Prepare the bacon to your liking and set aside. Combine the eggs, parmesan cheese, and your choice of finely chopped herbs. Warm a skillet and add the butter/ghee to melt using the medium-high heat setting. When the pan is hot, whisk and add the eggs.

2. Prepare the omelet working it towards the middle of the pan for about 30 seconds. When firm, flip, and cook it for another 30 seconds. Arrange the omelet on a plate and garnish with the crunched bacon bits. Serve with sliced avocado.

BACON & CHEESE FRITTATA

PREPARATION
5 MINS

COOKING
5 MINS

6 SERVINGS

INGREDIENTS

- 1 cup Heavy cream

- 6 Eggs

- 5 Crispy slices of bacon

- 2 Chopped green onions

- 4 oz Cheddar cheese

- Also Needed: 1 pie plate

NUTRIRION

- Carbohydrates: 2 grams

- Protein: 13 grams

- Fats: 29 grams

- Calories: 320

DIRECTIONS

1. Warm the oven temperature to reach 350° Fahrenheit.

2. Whisk the eggs and seasonings. Empty into the pie pan and top off with the remainder of the fixings. Bake 30-35 minutes. Wait for a few minutes before serving for best results

Bacon & Egg Breakfast Muffins

PREPARATION
15 MINS

COOKING
30 MINS

SERVINGS
12

INGREDIENTS

- 8 large Eggs

- 8 slices Bacon

- .66 cup Green onion

NUTRIRION

- Carbohydrates: 0.4 grams

- Protein: 5.6 grams

- Fats: 4.9 grams

- Calories: 69

DIRECTIONS

1. Warm the oven at 350° Fahrenheit. Spritz the muffin tin wells using a cooking oil spray. Chop the onions and set aside.

2. Prepare a large skillet using the medium temperature setting. Fry the bacon until it's crispy and place on a layer of paper towels to drain the grease. Chop it into small pieces after it has cooled.

3. Whisk the eggs, bacon, and green onions, mixing well until all of the fixings are incorporated. Dump the egg mixture into the muffin tin (halfway full). Bake it for about 20 to 25 minutes. Cool slightly and serve.

Bacon Hash

PREPARATION
5 MINS

COOKING
10 MINS

SERVINGS
2

INGREDIENTS

- Ingredients:

- 1 Small green pepper

- 2 Jalapenos

- 1 Small onion

- 4 Eggs

- 6 Bacon slices

NUTRIRION

- Carbohydrates: 9 grams

- Protein: 23 grams

- Fats: 24 grams

- Calories: 366

DIRECTIONS

1. Chop the bacon into chunks using a food processor. Set aside for now. Slice the onions and peppers into thin strips. Dice the jalapenos as small as possible.

2. Heat a skillet and fry the veggies. Once browned, combine the fixings and cook until crispy. Place on a serving dish with the eggs

Bagels With Cheese

PREPARATION
10 MINS

COOKING
15 MINS

SERVINGS
6

INGREDIENTS

- 2.5 cups Mozzarella cheese
- 1.5 cups Almond flour
- 1 tsp. Baking powder
- 2 Eggs
- 3 oz Cream cheese

NUTRIRION

- Carbohydrates: 8 grams
- Fats: 31 grams
- Protein: 19 grams
- Calories: 374

DIRECTIONS

1. Shred the mozzarella and combine with the flour, baking powder, and cream cheese in a mixing container. Pop into the microwave for about one minute. Mix well.

2. Let the mixture cool and add the eggs. Break apart into six sections and shape into round bagels. Note: You can also sprinkle with a seasoning of your choice or pinch of salt if desired.

3. Bake them for approximately 12 to 15 minutes. Serve or cool and store

BAKED APPLES

PREPARATION
10 MINS

COOKING
1 HOUR

SERVINGS
4

INGREDIENTS

- 4 tsp Keto-friendly sweetener.
- 75 tsp Cinnamon
- .25 cup chopped pecans
- 4 large Granny Smith apples

NUTRIRION

- Carbohydrates: 16 grams
- Protein: 6.8 grams
- Fats: 19.9 grams
- Calories: 175

DIRECTIONS

1. Set the oven temperature at 375° Fahrenheit. Mix the sweetener with the cinnamon and pecans. Core the apple and add the prepared stuffing.

2. Add enough water into the baking dish to cover the bottom of the apple. Bake them for about 45 minutes to 1 hour

Baked Eggs In The Avocado

PREPARATION
10 MINS

COOKING
20 MINS

SERVINGS
1

INGREDIENTS

- Half of 1 Avocado

- 1 Egg

- 1 tbsp Olive oil

- Half cup shredded cheddar cheese

NUTRIRION

- Carbohydrates: 3 grams

- Protein: 21 grams

- Fats: 52 grams

- Calories: 452

DIRECTIONS

1. Heat the oven to reach 425° Fahrenheit.

2. Discard the avocado pit and remove just enough of the 'insides' to add the egg. Drizzle with oil and break the egg into the shell.

3. Sprinkle with cheese and bake them for 15 to 16 minutes until the egg is the way you prefer. Serve.

Banana Pancakes

PREPARATION
10 MINS

COOKING
15 MINS

SERVINGS
3

INGREDIENTS

- 2 Bananas

- 4 Eggs

- 1 tsp Cinnamon

- 1 tsp Baking powder (Optional

NUTRIRION

- Carbohydrates: 6.8 grams

- Total: 7 grams

- Calories: 157

DIRECTIONS

1. Combine each of the fixings. Melt a portion of butter in a skillet using the medium temperature setting.

2. Prepare the pancakes 1-2 minutes per side. Cook them with the lid on for the first part of the cooking cycle for a fluffier pancake.

3. Serve plain or with your favorite garnishes such as a dollop of coconut cream or fresh berries

Breakfast Skillet

PREPARATION
10 MINS

COOKING
15 MINS

SERVINGS
2

INGREDIENTS

- 1 lb. Organic ground turkey/ grass-fed beef

- 6 Organic eggs

- 1 cup Keto-friendly salsa of choice

NUTRIRION

- Carbohydrates: 3 grams

- Protein: 21 grams

- Fats: 52 grams

- Calories: 452

DIRECTIONS

1. Warm the skillet using oil (medium heat). Add the turkey and simmer until the pink is gone. Fold in the salsa and simmer for two to three minutes.

2. Crack the eggs and add to the top of the turkey base. Place a lid on the pot and cook for seven minutes until the whites of the eggs are opaque.

3. Note: The cooking time will vary depending on how you like the eggs prepared

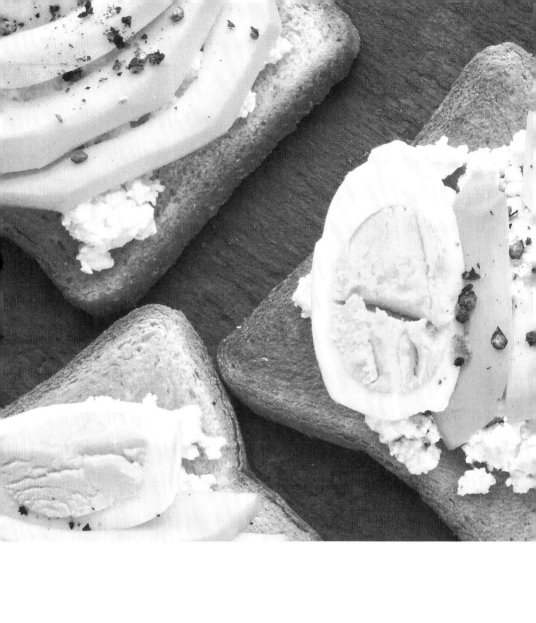

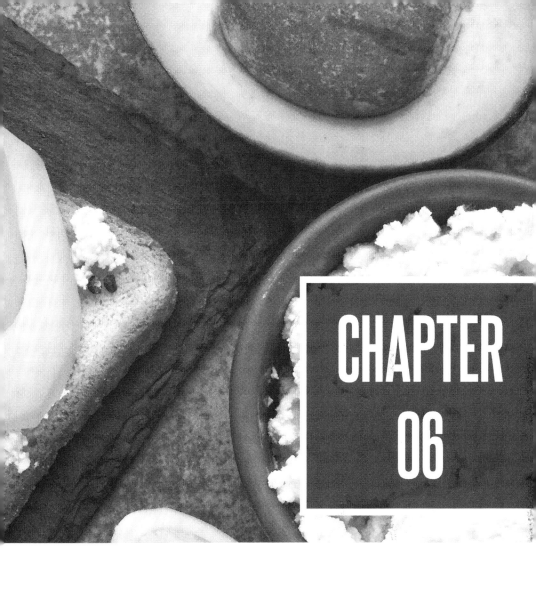

CHAPTER 06

APPETIZERS AND SIDE DISHES

Simple Kimchi

PREPARATION
10 MINS

COOKING
70 MINS

SERVINGS
4

INGREDIENTS

- 3 tablespoons salt

- 1 pound napa cabbage, chopped

- 1 carrot, julienned

- ½ cup daikon radish

- 3 green onion stalks, chopped

- 1 tablespoon fish sauce

- 3 tablespoons chili flakes

- 3 garlic cloves, peeled and minced

- 1 tablespoon sesame oil

- ½-inch fresh ginger, peeled and grated

NUTRIRION

- Calories: 160

- Fat: 3g

- Fiber: 2g

- Carbohydrates: 5g

- Protein: 1g

DIRECTIONS

1. In a bowl, mix the cabbage with the salt, massage well for 10 minutes, cover, and set aside for 1 hour.

2. In a bowl, mix the chili flakes with fish sauce, garlic, sesame oil, and ginger, and stir well.

3. Drain the cabbage well, rinse under cold water, and transfer to a bowl.

4. Add the carrots, green onions, radish, and chili paste and stir.

5. Leave in a dark and cold place for at least 2 days before serving.

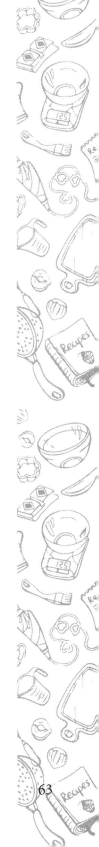

Oven-fried Green Beans

PREPARATION
10 MINS

COOKING
10 MINS

SERVINGS
4

INGREDIENTS

- Ingredients:

- ⅔ Cup Parmesan cheese, grated

- 1 egg

- 12 ounces green beans

- Salt and ground black pepper, to taste

- ½ teaspoon garlic powder

- ¼ teaspoon paprika

DIRECTIONS

1. In a bowl, mix the Parmesan cheese with salt, pepper, garlic powder, and paprika.

2. In another bowl, whisk the egg with salt and pepper. Dredge the green beans in egg, and then in the Parmesan mixture. Place the green beans on a lined baking sheet, place in an oven at 400°F for 10 minutes.

3. Serve hot.

NUTRIRION

- Calories: 114

- Fat: 5g

- Fiber: 7g

- Carbohydrates: 3g

- Protein: 9g

Cauliflower Mash

PREPARATION
10 MINS

COOKING
10 MINS

SERVINGS
2

INGREDIENTS

- ¼ cup sour cream

- 1 small cauliflower head, separated into florets

- Salt and ground black pepper, to taste

- 2 tablespoons feta cheese, crumbled

- 2 tablespoons black olives, pitted and sliced

DIRECTIONS

1. Put water in a pot, add some salt, bring to a boil over medium heat, add the florets, cook for 10 minutes, take off the heat, and drain.

2. Return the cauliflower to the pot, add salt, black pepper, and sour cream, and blend using an immersion blender.

3. Add the black olives and feta cheese, stir and serve.

NUTRIRION

- Calories: 100

- Fat: 4g

- Fiber: 2g

- Carbohydrates: 3g

- Protein: 2g

Portobello Mushrooms

PREPARATION
10 MINS

COOKING
10 MINS

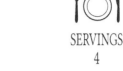

SERVINGS
4

INGREDIENTS

- T12 ounces Portobello mushrooms, sliced

- Salt and ground black pepper, to taste

- ½ teaspoon dried basil

- 2 tablespoons olive oil

- ½ teaspoon tarragon, dried

- ½ teaspoon dried rosemary

- ½ teaspoon dried thyme

- 2 tablespoons balsamic vinegar

DIRECTIONS

1. In a bowl, mix the oil with vinegar, salt, pepper, rosemary, tarragon, basil, and thyme, and whisk.

2. Add the mushroom slices, toss to coat well, place them on a pre-heated grill over medium-high heat, cook for 5 minutes on both sides, and serve.

NUTRIRION

- Calories: 280

- Fat: 4g

- Fiber: 4g

- Carbohydrates: 2g

- Protein: 4g

Broiled Brussels Sprouts

PREPARATION
10 MINS

COOKING
10 MINS

SERVINGS
4

INGREDIENTS

- 1 pound Brussels sprouts, trimmed and halved

- Salt and ground black pepper, to taste

- 1 teaspoon sesame seeds

- 1 tablespoon green onions, chopped

- 1½ tablespoons sukrin gold syrup

- 1 tablespoon coconut aminos

- 2 tablespoons sesame oil

- 1 tablespoon sriracha

DIRECTIONS

1. In a bowl, mix the sesame oil with coconut aminos, sriracha, syrup, salt, and black pepper, and whisk.

2. Heat a pan over medium-high heat, add the Brussels sprouts, and cook them for 5 minutes on each side.

3. Add the sesame oil mixture, toss to coat, sprinkle sesame seeds, and green onions, stir again, and serve

NUTRIRION

- Calories: 110

- Fat: 4g

- Fiber: 4g

- Carbohydrates: 6

- Protein: 4g

PESTO

PREPARATION
10 MINS

COOKING
0 MINS

SERVINGS
4

INGREDIENTS

- ½ cup olive oil

- 2 cups basil

- ⅓ cup pine nuts

- ⅓ cup Parmesan cheese,

grated

- 2 garlic cloves, peeled and chopped

- Salt and ground black pepper, to taste

DIRECTIONS

1. Put the basil in a food processor, add the pine nuts, and garlic, and blend well. Add the Parmesan cheese, salt, pepper, and the oil gradually and blend again until you obtain a paste. Serve with chicken or vegetables.

NUTRIRION

- Calories: 100

- Fat: 7g

- Fiber: 3g

- Carbohydrates: 1g

- Protein: 5g

Brussels Sprouts and Bacon

PREPARATION
10 MINS

COOKING
30 MINS

SERVINGS
4

INGREDIENTS

- 18 bacon strips, chopped

- 1 pound Brussels sprouts, trimmed and halved

- Salt and ground black pepper, to taste

- A pinch of cumin

- A pinch of red pepper, crushed

- 2 tablespoons extra virgin olive oil

DIRECTIONS

1. In a bowl, mix the Brussels sprouts with salt, pepper, cumin, red pepper, and oil, and toss to coat.

2. Spread the Brussels sprouts on a lined baking sheet, place in an oven at 375°F, and bake for 30 minutes.

3. Heat a pan over medium heat, add the bacon pieces, and cook them until they become crispy.

4. Divide the baked Brussels sprouts on plates, top with bacon, and serve.

NUTRIRION

- Calories: 256

- Fat: 20g

- Fiber: 6g

- Carbohydrates: 5g

- Protein: 15g

CREAMY SPINACH

PREPARATION
10 MINS

COOKING
15 MINS

SERVINGS
2

INGREDIENTS

- 2 garlic cloves, peeled and minced

- 8 ounces of spinach leaves

- A drizzle of olive oil

- Salt and ground black pepper, to taste

- 4 tablespoons sour cream

- 1 tablespoon butter

- 2 tablespoons Parmesan cheese, grated

DIRECTIONS

1. Heat a pan with the oil over medium heat, add the spinach, stir and cook until it softens.

2. Add the salt, pepper, butter, Parmesan cheese, and butter, stir, and cook for 4 minutes.

3. Add the sour cream, stir, and cook for 5 minutes.

4. Divide between plates and serve

NUTRIRION

- Calories: 233

- Fat: 10g

- Fiber: 4g

- Carbohydrates: 4g

- Protein: 2g

Avocado Fries

PREPARATION
10 MINS

COOKING
5 MINS

SERVINGS
3

INGREDIENTS

- 3 avocados, pitted, peeled, halved, and sliced

- 1½ cups sunflower oil

- 1½ cups almond meal

- A pinch of cayenne pepper

- Salt and ground black pepper, to taste

DIRECTIONS

1. In a bowl, mix the almond meal with salt, pepper, and cayenne, and stir. In a second bowl, whisk eggs with a pinch of salt and pepper.

2. Dredge the avocado pieces in egg and then in almond meal mixture. Heat a pan with the oil over medium-high heat, add the avocado fries, and cook them until they are golden.

3. Transfer to paper towels, drain grease, and divide between plates and serve.

NUTRIRION

- Calories: 200

- Fat: 43g

- Fiber: 4g

- Carbs: 7g

- Protein: 17g

ROASTED CAULIFLOWER

PREPARATION
10 MINS

COOKING
25 MINS

SERVINGS
6

INGREDIENTS

- 1 cauliflower head, separated into florets

- Salt and ground black pepper, to taste

- ⅓ cup Parmesan cheese, grated

- 1 tablespoon fresh parsley, chopped

- 3 tablespoons olive oil

- 2 tablespoons extra virgin olive oil

DIRECTIONS

1. In a bowl, mix the oil with garlic, salt, pepper, and cauliflower florets.

2. Toss to coat well, spread this on a lined baking sheet, place in an oven at 450°F, and bake for 25 minutes, stirring halfway. Add the Parmesan cheese, and parsley, stir and cook for 5 minutes.

3. Divide between plates and serve.

NUTRIRION

- Calories: 118

- Fat: 2g

- Fiber: 3g

- Carbohydrates: 2g

- Protein: 6g

MUSHROOMS AND SPINACH

PREPARATION
10 MINS

COOKING
10 MINS

SERVINGS
4

INGREDIENTS

- 10 ounces spinach leaves, chopped
- Salt and ground black pepper, to taste
- 14 ounces mushrooms, chopped
- 2 garlic cloves, peeled and minced
- ½ cup fresh parsley, chopped
- 1 onion, peeled and chopped
- 4 tablespoons olive oil
- 2 tablespoons balsamic vinegar

DIRECTIONS

1. Heat a pan with the oil over medium-high heat, add the garlic and onion, stir, and cook for 4 minutes.

2. Add the mushrooms, stir, and cook for 3 minutes.

3. Add the spinach, stir, and cook for 3 minutes.

4. Add the vinegar, salt, and pepper, stir, and cook for 1 minute.

5. Add the parsley, stir, divide between plates, and serve.

NUTRIRION

- Calories: 200
- Fat: 4g
- Fiber: 6g
- Carbohydrates: 2g
- Protein: 12g

Collard Greens with Turkey

PREPARATION
10 MINS

COOKING
135 MINS

SERVINGS
10

INGREDIENTS

- 5 bunches collard greens, chopped

- Salt and ground black pepper, to taste

- 1 tablespoon red pepper flakes

- 5 cups chicken stock

- 1 turkey leg

- 2 tablespoons garlic, minced

- ¼ cup olive oil

DIRECTIONS

1. Heat a pot with the oil over medium heat, add the garlic, stir, and cook for 1 minute.

2. Add the stock, salt, pepper, and turkey leg stir, cover, and simmer for 30 minutes.

3. Add the collard greens, cover pot again, and cook for 45 minutes.

4. Reduce heat to medium, add more salt and pepper, stir, and cook for 1 hour.

5. Drain the greens, chop up the turkey, mix everything with the red pepper flakes, stir, divide between plates, and serve.

NUTRIRION

- Calories: 143
- Fat: 3g
- Fiber: 4g

- Carbohydrates: 3g
- Protein: 6g

Eggplant and Tomatoes

PREPARATION
10 MINS

COOKING
10 MINS

SERVINGS
4

INGREDIENTS

- 1 tomato, sliced

- 1 eggplant, sliced into thin rounds

- Salt and ground black pepper, to taste

- ¼ cup Parmesan cheese, grated

- A drizzle of olive oil

DIRECTIONS

1. Place eggplant slices on a lined baking dish, drizzle some oil and sprinkle half of the Parmesan.

2. Top eggplant slices with tomato ones, season with some salt and pepper, and sprinkle the rest of the cheese over them.

3. Place in an oven at 400°F, and bake for 15 minutes.

4. Divide between plates and serve hot as a side dish.

NUTRIRION

- Calories: 55

- Fat: 1.1g

- Fiber: 2g

- Carbohydrates: 0.5g

- Protein: 7g

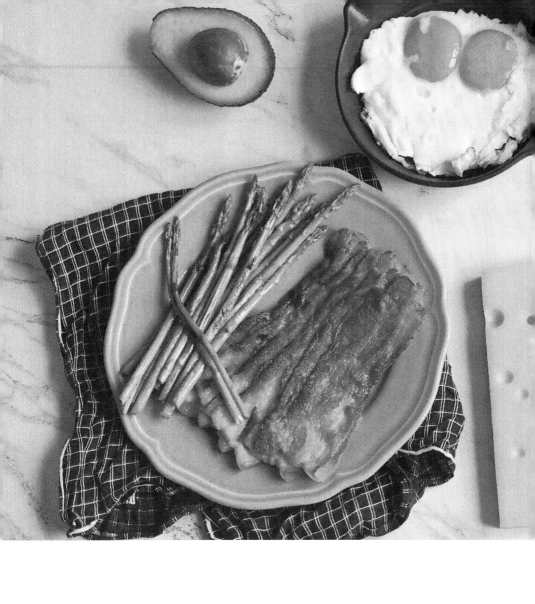

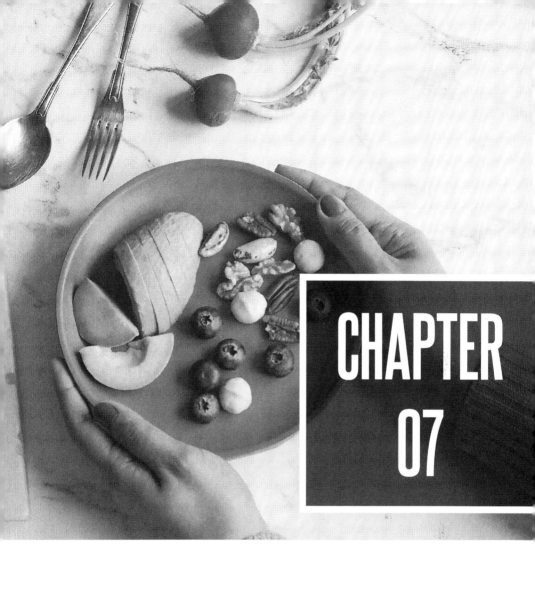

LUNCH

Taco Stuffed Avocados

PREPARATION
12 MINS

COOKING
18 MINS

SERVINGS
6

INGREDIENTS

- 4 Ripe Avocados

- Juice of 1 Lime

- 1 Tbsp. Extra-Virgin Olive Oil

- 1 Medium Onion, Chopped

- 1 Lb. Ground Beef

- 1 Packet Taco Seasoning

- Kosher Salt

- Freshly Ground Black Pepper

- 2/3 Cup Shredded Mexican Cheese

- 1/2 Cup Shredded Lettuce

- 1/2 Cup Quartered Grape Tomatoes

- Sour cream, for topping

NUTRIRION

- Calories: 352

- Carbohydrates: 3.6g

- Fat: 27.4g

- Protein: 22.4g

DIRECTIONS

1. Pit and halve the avocados.

2. With a scoop, scoop out a bit of avocado flesh to create a hole.

3. Dice the removed avocado fresh and set aside for later.

4. Pour lime juice over the avocados to prevent browning.

5. Heat oil in a preheated skillet over medium heat and add chopped onion.

6. Cook the onion until translucent for 3-5 minutes.

7. Stir in ground beef and taco seasoning, breaking up the meat with a wooden spoon.

8. Season the beef with salt and pepper, cook until the meat is browned and no longer pink, about 6 minutes.

9. Turn off the heat and drain the fat, top each avocado half with the cooked beef mixture.

10. Then top with chopped avocado, cheese, lettuce, tomato, and sour cream.

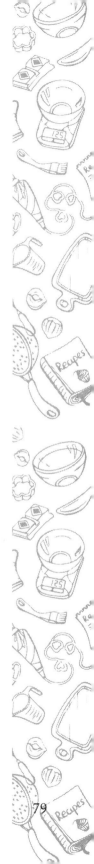

Buffalo Shrimp Lettuce Wraps

PREPARATION
17 MINS

COOKING
23 MINS

SERVINGS
4

INGREDIENTS

- 1/4 Tbsp. Butter

- 2 Garlic Cloves, Minced

- 1/4 C. Hot Sauce, Such as Frank's

- 1 Tbsp. Extra-Virgin Olive Oil

- 1 Lb. Shrimp, Peeled and Deveined, Tails Removed

- Kosher Salt

- Freshly Ground Black Pepper

- 1 Head Romaine lettuce, Leaves Separated, For Serving

- 1/4 Red Onion, Finely Chopped

- 1 Rib Celery, Sliced Thin

- 1/2 C. Blue Cheese, Crumble

NUTRIRION

- Calories: 190

- Carbohydrates: 6g

- Fat: 9.3g

- Protein: 18.1g

DIRECTIONS

1. Pit and halve the avocados.

2. With a scoop, scoop out a bit of avocado flesh to create a hole.

3. Dice the removed avocado fresh and set aside for later.

4. Pour lime juice over the avocados to prevent browning.

5. Heat oil in a preheated skillet over medium heat and add chopped onion.

6. Cook the onion until translucent for 3-5 minutes.

7. Stir in ground beef and taco seasoning, breaking up the meat with a wooden spoon.

8. Season the beef with salt and pepper, cook until the meat is browned and no longer pink, about 6 minutes.

9. Turn off the heat and drain the fat, top each avocado half with the cooked beef mixture.

10. Then top with chopped avocado, cheese, lettuce, tomato, and sour cream

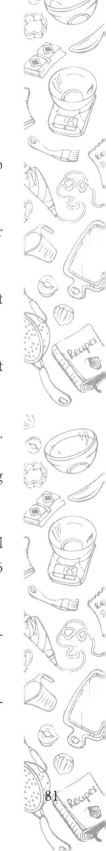

KETO BACON SUSHI

PREPARATION
13 MINS

COOKING
20 MINS

SERVINGS
12

INGREDIENTS

- 6 slices bacon, halved

- 2 Persian cucumbers, thinly sliced

- 2 medium carrots, thinly sliced

- 1 avocado, sliced

- 4 oz. cream cheese softened

- Sesame seeds, for garnish

NUTRIRION

- Calories: 155

- Carbohydrates: 6.7g

- Fat: 12.7g

- Protein: 4.4 g

DIRECTIONS

1. Heat oven to 400 °F (204 °C), line a baking tray with aluminum foil and fit it with a cooling rack.

2. Lay bacon halves in an even layer on the lined baking sheet and place in the oven.

3. Bake until lightly crunchy but still pliable, about 11 to 13 minutes.

4. In the meantime, cut cucumbers, carrots, and avocado into pieces roughly the width of the bacon.

5. Once the bacon is cool enough to touch, spread an even layer of cream cheese on each slice.

6. Divide vegetables evenly between the bacon and place on one end.

7. Roll up vegetables tightly.

8. Garnish with sesame seeds and serve.

9. Enjoy.

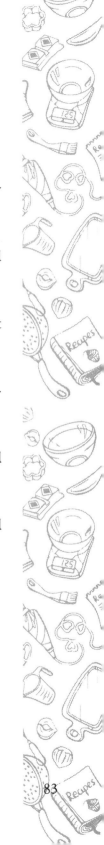

Keto Burger Fat Bombs

PREPARATION
12 MINS

COOKING
15 MINS

SERVINGS
20

INGREDIENTS

- Cooking spray

- 1 lb. ground beef

- 1/2 tsp. garlic powder

- Kosher salt

- Freshly ground black pepper

- 2 tbsp. cold butter, cut into 20 pieces

- 2 oz. cheddar, cut into 20 pieces

- Lettuce leaves, for serving

- Thinly sliced tomatoes, for serving

- Mustard, for serving

NUTRIRION

- Calories: 77.5

- Carbohydrates: 1.7g

- Fat: 4.8g

- Protein: 6.3g

DIRECTIONS

1. Heat oven to 375 °F (190 °C), grease a mini muffin tin with cooking spray.

2. In a medium bowl, season beef with garlic powder, salt, and pepper.

3. Press one teaspoon beef consistently into the bottom of each muffin tin cup, totally covering the bottom.

4. Place a slice of butter on top then press one teaspoon beef over butter to cover.

5. Place a slice of cheddar on top of meat in each cup then press remaining beef over cheese to cover.

6. Bake the fat bombs until meat is golden and cook through for about 15 minutes.

7. Let cool slightly.

8. Carefully, use a metal offset spatula to release each burger from the tin. Serve with lettuce leaves, tomatoes, and mustard.

9. Enjoy

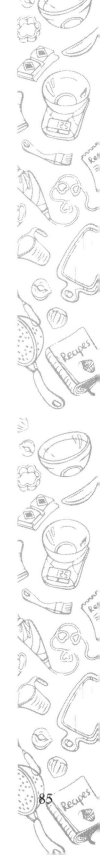

KETO TACO CUPS

PREPARATION
12 MINS

COOKING
20 MINS

SERVINGS
12

INGREDIENTS

- 2 C. Shredded Cheddar

- 1 Tbsp. Extra-Virgin Olive Oil

- 1 Small Onion, Chopped

- 3 Cloves Garlic, Minced

- 1 Lb. Ground Beef

- 1 Tsp. Chili Powder

- 1/2 Tsp. Ground Cumin

- 1/2 Tsp. Paprika

- Kosher salt

- Freshly ground black pepper

- Sour cream, for serving

- Diced avocado, for serving

- Freshly chopped cilantro, for serving

- Chopped tomatoes, for serving

NUTRIRION

- Calories: 189.8

- Carbohydrates: 1.1g

- Fat: 14.2g

- Protein: 14.2g

DIRECTIONS

1. Preheat oven to 375 °F (190 °C).

2. Line a large baking tray with parchment paper or a baking mat.

3. Put about 2 tablespoons cheddar with a space of 2-inches.

4. Bake the cheese until bubbly and edges turn to golden, about 5-7 minutes.

5. Let the crisps cool on the baking sheet for a minute.

6. Grease bottom of a muffin tin with cooking spray set aside.

7. Put the backed melted cheese slices on the bottom of a muffin tin.

8. Top with another muffin tin and let it cool for 8-10 minutes.

9. Heat oil in a skillet over medium heat, add chopped onion and cook until soft.

10. Add garlic and cook until fragrant, add ground beef, breaking up meat with a spatula.

11. Cook until beef is browned and no longer pink, about 4-6 minutes, then drain the fat.

12. Add meat again to the skillet and season with chili powder, cumin, paprika, salt, and pepper.

13. Place cheese cups on a serving platter.

14. Fill the cheese cups with cooked ground beef and top with sour cream, avocado, cilantro, and tomatoes.

15. Enjoy

CAPRESE ZOODLES

PREPARATION
25 MINS

COOKING
0 MINS

SERVINGS
4

INGREDIENTS

- 4 Large Zucchini

- 2 Tbsp. Extra-Virgin Olive Oil

- Kosher Salt

- Freshly Ground Black Pepper

- 2 C. Cherry Tomatoes Halved

- 1 C. Mozzarella Balls, Quartered If Large

- 1/4 C. Fresh Basil Leaves

- 2 Tbsp. Balsamic Vinegar

NUTRIRION

- Calories: 311
- Carbohydrates: 7.4g

- Fat: 22.2g
- Protein: 16.7g

DIRECTIONS

1. Using a spiralizer, make zoodles out of zucchini.

2. Put zoodles to a big bowl, toss with olive oil and season with pepper and salt.

3. Let marinate 15 minutes.

4. Combine in tomatoes, mozzarella, and basil to zoodles in a bowl and toss until combined.

5. Drizzle with balsamic and serve.

6. Enjoy

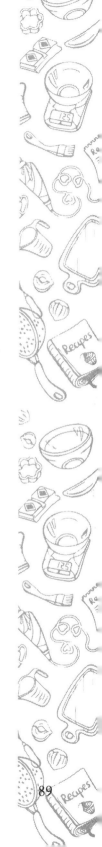

Zucchini Sushi

PREPARATION
20 MINS

COOKING
0 MINS

SERVINGS
2

INGREDIENTS

- 2 medium zucchini

- 4 oz. cream cheese softened

- 1 tsp. Sriracha hot sauce

- 1 tsp. lime juice

- 1 c. lump crab meat

- 1/2 carrot, cut into thin

matchsticks

- 1/2 avocado, diced

- 1/2 cucumber, cut into thin matchsticks

- 1 tsp. toasted sesame seeds

NUTRIRION

- Calories: 378.8

- Carbohydrates: 10.5g

- Fat: 25.5g

- Protein: 27.7g

DIRECTIONS

1. With a vegetable peeler, slice each zucchini into even thin strips.

2. Place zucchini on a lined plate to dry up the moisture.

3. In a bowl, whisk together cream cheese, Sriracha, and lime juice.

4. Place two zucchini slices down straight on a cutting board.

5. Top with cream cheese in a thin layer on the lift side top with crab, cucumber, and avocado.

6. Roll the zucchini tightly from the lift side.

7. Repeat the process with the remaining zucchini pieces.

8. Garnish with sesame seeds before serving.

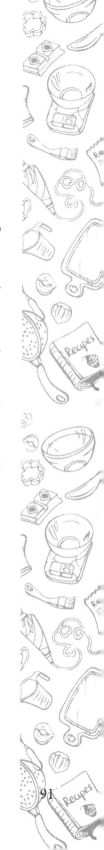

ASIAN CHICKEN LETTUCE WRAPS

PREPARATION
13 MINS

COOKING
15 MINS

SERVINGS
4

INGREDIENTS

- 3 tbsp. hoisin sauce

- 2 tbsp. low-sodium soy sauce

- 2 tbsp. rice wine vinegar

- 1 tbsp. Sriracha (optional)

- 1 tsp. sesame oil

- 1 tbsp. extra-virgin olive oil

- 1 medium onion, diced

- 2 cloves garlic, minced

- 1 tbsp. freshly grated ginger

- 1 lb. ground chicken

- 1/2 c. water chestnuts, drained and sliced

- 2 green onions, thinly sliced

- Kosher salt

- Freshly ground black pepper

- Large leafy lettuce (leaves separated), for serving

-

NUTRIRION

- Calories: 280.85

- Carbohydrates: 8.7g

- Fat: 17.6g

- Protein: 21.4g

DIRECTIONS

1. Make the sauce: In a thin bowl.

2. Whisk together hoisin sauce, rice wine vinegar, soy sauce, Sriracha, and sesame oil.

3. In a big skillet over medium-high heat, preheat olive oil.

4. Put onions and cook until soft, about 5 minutes.

5. Then stir in garlic and ginger and cook until fragrant, about 1 minute more.

6. Put ground chicken and cook until opaque and typically cooked through, breaking up meat with a wooden spoon.

7. Pour in the sauce and cook 1 to 2 minutes more, until sauce reduces slightly and chicken cooked through thoroughly.

8. Turn off heat and stir in chestnuts and green onions.

9. Season with pepper and salt.

10. Spoon rice, if using, and a large scoop (about 1/4 cup) of chicken mixture into the center of each lettuce leaf. Serve immediately

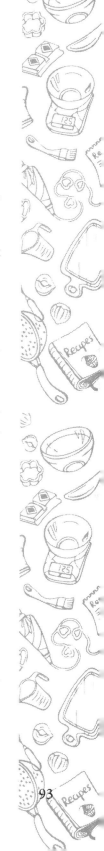

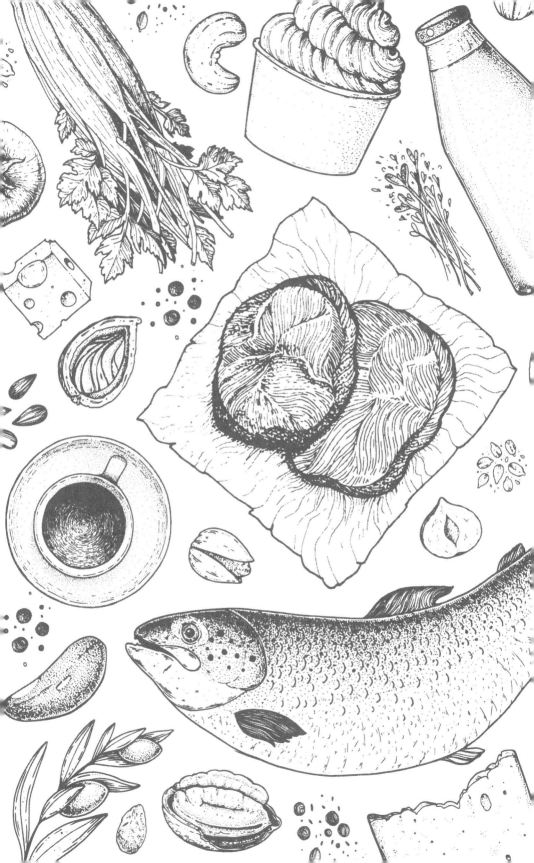

Prosciutto and Mozzarella Bomb

PREPARATION
11 MINS

COOKING
15 MINS

SERVINGS
4

INGREDIENTS

- 4 oz (113g) sliced prosciutto

- 8 oz (226g) fresh mozzarella ball

- Olive oil, for frying

-

DIRECTIONS

1. Coating half of the prosciutto slices vertically.

2. Lay the remaining slices horizontally across the first set of slices.

3. Place your mozzarella ball, upside down, onto the crisscrossed prosciutto slices.

4. Firmly, but very carefully, wrap the mozzarella ball with the prosciutto slices.

5. If making ahead, wrap the balls in cling film and refrigerate.

6. To serve, heat the olive oil in a skillet and crisp the prosciutto on all sides

NUTRIRION

- Calories: 129
- Carbohydrates: 0.3g

- Fat: 11.6g
- Protein: 6.2g

Ketofied Chick-Fil-A-style Chicken

PREPARATION
14 MINS

COOKING
21 MINS

SERVINGS
8

INGREDIENTS

- 24-oz (680g) pickle jar

- 8 medium uncooked chicken breast tenders

- 4 tbsp almond flour

- ¼ cup grated Parmesan

- Salt and pepper, to taste

- 1 tsp paprika

- 2 large eggs

- 2 tbsp avocado oil

NUTRIRION

- Calories: 407

- Carbohydrates: 12.5g

- Fat: 23.6g

- Protein: 28g

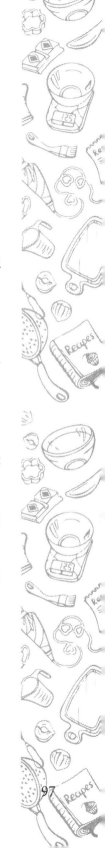

DIRECTIONS

1. In a plastic resealable bag, add the chicken and the pickle juice, marinate in the fridge

2. For 20-30 minutes.

3. On a plate combine the almond flour, grated Parmesan, salt, pepper, and paprika.

4. Whip the eggs together in a separate bowl.

5. Preheat a skillet over medium-high heat and heat the avocado oil.

6. First, dip the chicken pieces in the beaten egg then place it in the breading mixture to coat.

7. Place the chicken into the skillet and cook until golden browned.

CHEESEBURGER TOMATOES

PREPARATION
7 MINS

COOKING
25 MINS

SERVINGS
4

INGREDIENTS

- 1 tbsp. extra-virgin olive oil
- 1 medium onion, chopped
- 2 cloves garlic, minced
- 1 lb. ground beef
- 1 tbsp. ketchup
- 1 tbsp. yellow mustard
- 4 slicing tomatoes

- Kosher salt
- Freshly ground black pepper
- 2/3 c. shredded cheddar
- 1/4 c. shredded iceberg lettuce
- 4 pickle coins
- Sesame seeds, for garnish

NUTRIRION

- Calories: 458
- Carbohydrates: 5g

- Fat: 32.8g
- Protein: 33.4g

DIRECTIONS

1. In a skillet over medium heat, heat oil.

2. Put onion and cook until tender, about 5 minutes, then stir in garlic.

3. Place ground beef, cook and break up the meat with a spatula, cook until the beef browned about 6 minutes, drain fat.

4. Season with salt and pepper, then add the ketch-up and mustard.

5. Flip tomatoes so they are stem-side down.

6. Cut the tomatoes into six wedges, being careful not to cut entirely through the tomatoes.

7. Carefully spread open the wedges.

8. Divide cooked ground beef evenly among the to-matoes.

9. Then top each with cheese and lettuce.

10. Garnish with pickle coins and sesame seeds.

11. Serve it and enjoy it!

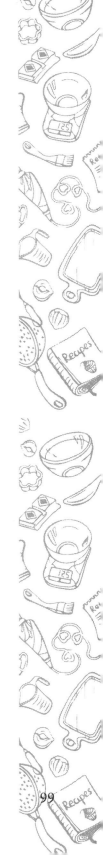

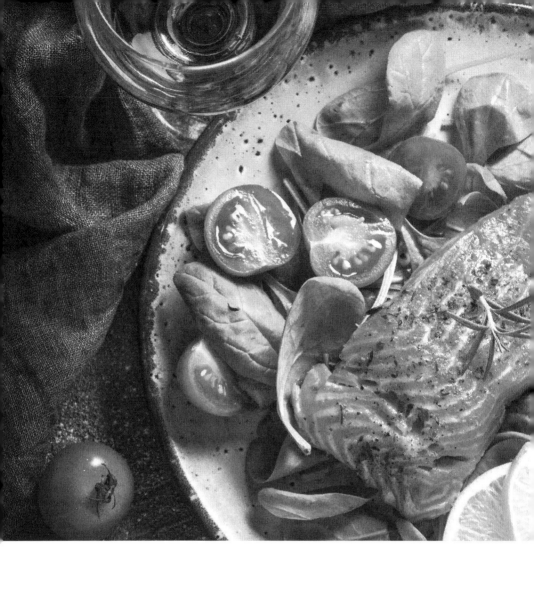

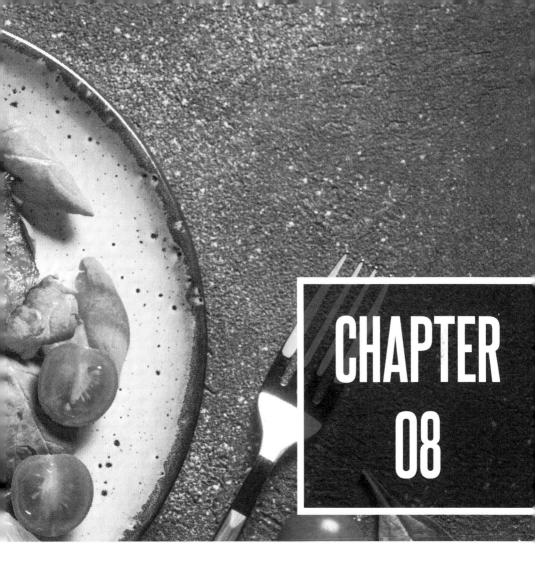

CHAPTER 08

DINNER

Korma Curry

PREPARATION
10 MINS

COOKING
25 MINS

SERVINGS
6

INGREDIENTS

- 3-pound chicken breast, skinless, boneless

- 1 teaspoon garam masala

- 1 teaspoon curry powder

- 1 tablespoon apple cider vinegar

- ½ coconut cream

- 1 cup organic almond milk

- 1 teaspoon ground coriander

- ¾ teaspoon ground cardamom

- ½ teaspoon ginger powder

- ¼ teaspoon cayenne pepper

- ¾ teaspoon ground cinnamon

- 1 tomato, diced

- 1 teaspoon avocado oil

- ½ cup of water

NUTRIRION

- Calories: 440

- Fat: 32g

- Fiber: 4g

- Carbohydrates: 28g

- Protein: 8g

DIRECTIONS

1. Chop the chicken breast and put it in the sauce-pan.

2. Add avocado oil and start to cook it over the medium heat.

3. Sprinkle the chicken with garam masala, curry powder, apple cider vinegar, ground coriander, cardamom, ginger powder, cayenne pepper, ground cinnamon, and diced tomato. Mix up the ingredients carefully. Cook them for 10 minutes.

4. Add water, coconut cream, and almond milk. Saute the meat for 10 minutes more

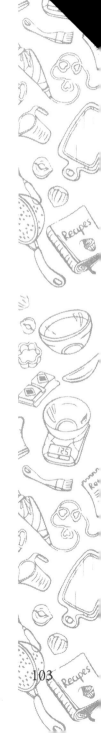

Zucchini Bars

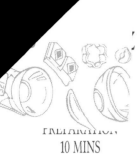

PREPARATION
10 MINS

COOKING
15 MINS

SERVINGS
8

INGREDIENTS

- 3 zucchini, grated
- ½ white onion, diced
- 2 teaspoons butter
- 3 eggs, whisked
- 4 tablespoons coconut flour
- 1 teaspoon salt
- ½ teaspoon ground black

pepper

- 5 oz goat cheese, crumbled
- 4 oz Swiss cheese, shredded
- ½ cup spinach, chopped
- 1 teaspoon baking powder
- ½ teaspoon lemon juice

NUTRIRION

- Calories: 187.2
- Total Fat: 7.3 g
- Saturated Fat: 0.6 g
- Cholesterol: 17.6 mg

- Sodium : 29.5 mg
- Potassium: 74.2 mg
- Total Carbohydrate: 29.5 g
- Protein: 1.7 g

DIRECTIONS

1. In the mixing bowl, mix up together grated zucchini, diced onion, eggs, coconut flour, salt, ground black pepper, crumbled cheese, chopped spinach, baking powder, and lemon juice.

2. Add butter and churn the mixture until homogenous.

3. Line the baking dish with baking paper.

4. Transfer the zucchini mixture into the baking dish and flatten it.

5. Preheat the oven to 365F and put the dish inside.

6. Cook it for 15 minutes. Then chill the meal well.

7. Cut it into bars.

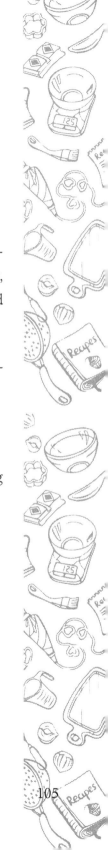

Mushroom Soup

PREPARATION
10 MINS

COOKING
25 MINS

SERVINGS
4

INGREDIENTS

- 1 cup of water

- 1 cup of coconut milk

- 1 cup white mushrooms, chopped

- ½ carrot, chopped

- ¼ white onion, diced

- 1 tablespoon butter

- 2 oz turnip, chopped

- 1 teaspoon dried dill

- ½ teaspoon ground black pepper

- ¾ teaspoon smoked paprika

- 1 oz celery stalk, chopped

NUTRIRION

- Calories: 39

- Total Fat: 2.6 g

- Cholesterol: 0 mg

- Sodium: 340 mg

- Potassium: 31 mg

- Total Carbohydrate: 3.3 g

- Protein: 0.7 g

DIRECTIONS

1. Pour water and coconut milk in the saucepan. Bring the liquid to boil.

2. Add chopped mushrooms, carrot, and turnip. Close the lid and boil for 10 minutes.

3. Meanwhile, put butter in the skillet. Add diced onion. Sprinkle it with dill, ground black pepper, and smoked paprika. Roast the onion for 3 minutes.

4. Add the roasted onion in the soup mixture.

5. Then add chopped celery stalk. Close the lid.

6. Cook soup for 10 minutes.

7. Then ladle it into the serving bowls.

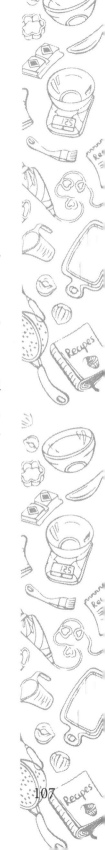

STUFFED PORTOBELLO MUSHROOMS

PREPARATION
10 MINS

COOKING
10 MINS

SERVINGS
4

INGREDIENTS

- 2 portobello mushrooms

- 1 cup spinach, chopped, steamed

- 2 oz artichoke hearts, drained, chopped

- 1 tablespoon coconut cream

- 1 tablespoon cream cheese

- 1 teaspoon minced garlic

- 1 tablespoon fresh cilantro, chopped

- 3 oz Cheddar cheese, grated

- ½ teaspoon ground black pepper

- 2 tablespoons olive oil

- ½ teaspoon salt

NUTRIRION

- Calories: 135.2

- Total Fat: 5.5 g

- Cholesterol: 16.4 mg

- Sodium : 698.1 mg

- Potassium: 275.3 mg

- Total Carbohydrate: 8.4 g

- Protein: 14.8 g

DIRECTIONS

1. Sprinkle mushrooms with olive oil and place in the tray.

2. Transfer the tray in the preheated to 360F oven and broil them for 5 minutes.

3. Meanwhile, blend artichoke hearts, coconut cream, cream cheese, minced garlic, and chopped cilantro.

4. Add grated cheese in the mixture and sprinkle with ground black pepper and salt.

5. Fill the broiled mushrooms with the cheese mixture and cook them for 5 minutes more. Serve the mushrooms only hot

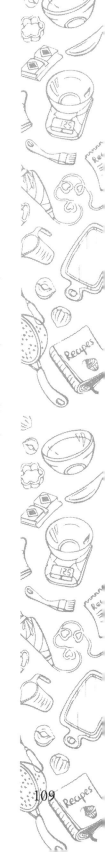

Lettuce Salad

PREPARATION
10 MINS

COOKING
0 MINS

SERVINGS
1

INGREDIENTS

- 1 cup Romaine lettuce, roughly chopped

- 3 oz seitan, chopped

- 1 tablespoon avocado oil

- 1 teaspoon sunflower seeds

- 1 teaspoon lemon juice

- 1 egg, boiled, peeled

- 2 oz Cheddar cheese, shredded

NUTRIRION

- Calories 20

- Total Fat 0.2g

- Cholesterol 0mg

- Sodium 31mg

- Potassium 241mg

- Total Carbohydrates 4.2g

- Protein 1.2g

DIRECTIONS

1. Place lettuce in the salad bowl. Add chopped seitan and shredded cheese.

2. Then chop the egg roughly and add in the salad bowl too.

3. Mix up together lemon juice with the avocado oil.

4. Sprinkle the salad with the oil mixture and sunflower seeds. Don't stir the salad before serving.

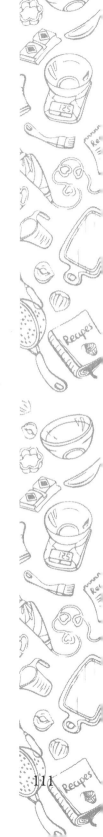

Onion Soup

PREPARATION
10 MINS

COOKING
25 MINS

SERVINGS
6

INGREDIENTS

- 2 cups white onion, diced

- 4 tablespoon butter

- ½ cup white mushrooms, chopped

- 3 cups of water

- 1 cup heavy cream

- 1 teaspoon salt

- 1 teaspoon chili flakes

- 1 teaspoon garlic powder

NUTRIRION

- Calories: 290.

- Fat: 9.6g.

- Protein: 16.8g.

- Carbohydrate: 33.4g.

DIRECTIONS

1. PPut butter in the saucepan and melt it.

2. Add diced white onion, chili flakes, and garlic powder. Mix it up and saute for 10 minutes over the medium-low heat.

3. Then add water, heavy cream, and chopped mushrooms. Close the lid.

4. Cook the soup for 15 minutes more.

5. Then blend the soup until you get the creamy texture. Ladle it in the bowls.

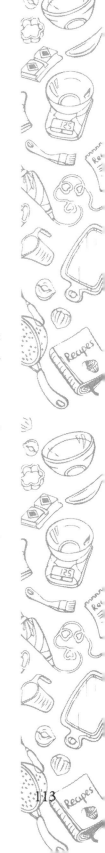

Asparagus Salad

PREPARATION
10 MINS

COOKING
15 MINS

SERVINGS
3

INGREDIENTS

- 10 oz asparagus

- 1 tablespoon olive oil

- ½ teaspoon white pepper

- 4 oz Feta cheese, crumbled

- 1 cup lettuce, chopped

- 1 tablespoon canola oil

- 1 teaspoon apple cider vinegar

- 1 tomato, diced

NUTRIRION

- Calories: 87.5

- Total Fat: 4.1 g

- Cholesterol: 9.2 mg

- Sodium: 685.8 mg

- Potassium: 212.1 mg

- Total Carbohydrate: 8.1 g

- Protein: 5.1 g

DIRECTIONS

1. SPreheat the oven to 365F.

2. Place asparagus in the tray, sprinkle with olive oil and white pepper and transfer in the preheated oven. Cook it for 15 minutes.

3. Meanwhile, put crumbled Feta in the salad bowl.

4. Add chopped lettuce and diced tomato.

5. Sprinkle the ingredients with apple cider vinegar.

6. Chill the cooked asparagus to the room temperature and add in the salad.

7. Shake the salad gently before serving.

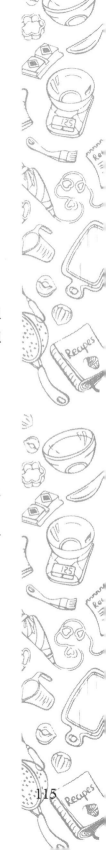

Beef with Cabbage Noodles

PREPARATION
5 MINS

COOKING
18 MINS

SERVINGS
2

INGREDIENTS

- 4 oz ground beef

- 1 cup chopped cabbage

- 4 oz tomato sauce

- ½ tsp minced garlic

- ½ cup of water

- Seasoning:

- ½ tbsp coconut oil

- ½ tsp salt

- ¼ tsp Italian seasoning

- 1/8 tsp dried basil

NUTRIRION

- Calories: 188.5

- Fats: 12.5 g

- Protein: 15.5 g

- Net Carbohydrates: 2.5 g

- Fiber: 1 g

DIRECTIONS

1. Take a skillet pan, place it over medium heat, add oil and when hot, add beef and cook for 5 minutes until nicely browned.

2. Meanwhile, prepare the cabbage and, for it, slice the cabbage into thin shred.

3. When the beef has cooked, add garlic, season with salt, basil, and Italian seasoning, stir well and continue cooking for 3 minutes until beef has thoroughly cooked.

4. Pour in tomato sauce and water, stir well and bring the mixture to boil.

5. Then reduce heat to medium-low level, add cabbage, stir well until well mixed and simmer for 3 to 5 minutes until cabbage is softened, covering the pan.

6. Uncover the pan and continue simmering the beef until most of the cooking liquid has evaporated.

7. Serve.

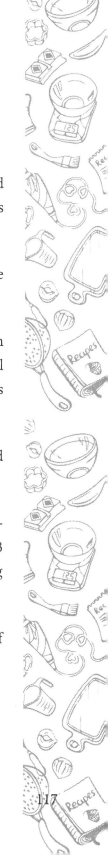

Roast Beef and Mozzarella Plate

PREPARATION
5 MINS

COOKING
0 MINS

SERVINGS
2

INGREDIENTS

- 4 slices of roast beef

- ½ ounce chopped lettuce

- 1 avocado, pitted

- 2 oz mozzarella cheese, cubed

- ½ cup mayonnaise

- Seasoning:

- ¼ tsp salt

- 1/8 tsp ground black pepper

- 2 tbsp avocado oil

NUTRIRION

- Calories: 267.7

- Fats: 24.5 g

- Protein: 9.5 g

- Net Carbohydrates: 1.5 g

- Fiber: 2 g

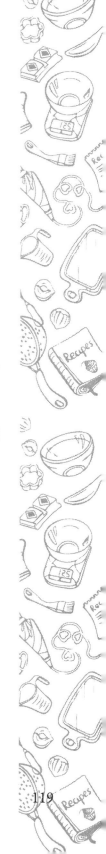

DIRECTIONS

1. Scoop out flesh from avocado and divide it evenly between two plates.

2. Add slices of roast beef, lettuce, and cheese and then sprinkle with salt and black pepper.

3. Serve with avocado oil and mayonnaise.

BEEF AND BROCCOLI

PREPARATION
5 MINS

COOKING
10 MINS

SERVINGS
2

INGREDIENTS

- 6 slices of beef roast, cut into strips

- 1 scallion, chopped

- 3 oz broccoli florets, chopped

- 1 tbsp avocado oil

- 1 tbsp butter, unsalted

- Seasoning:

- ¼ tsp salt

- 1/8 tsp ground black pepper

- 1 ½ tbsp soy sauce

- 3 tbsp chicken broth

NUTRIRION

- Calories: 15.7 g

- Fats: 21.6 g

- Protein: 1.7 g

- Net Carbohydrates:1.3 g

DIRECTIONS

1. Take a medium skillet pan, place it over medium heat, add oil and when hot, add beef strips and cook for 2 minutes until hot.

2. Transfer beef to a plate, add scallion to the pan, then add butter and cook for 3 minutes until tender.

3. Add remaining ingredients, stir until mixed, switch heat to the low level, and simmer for 3 to 4 minutes until broccoli is tender.

4. Return beef to the pan, stir until well combined and cook for 1 minute.

5. Serve

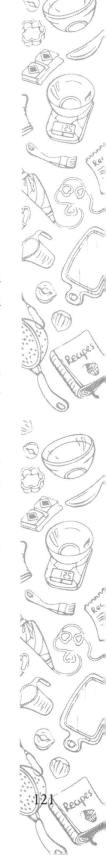

Garlic Herb Beef Roast

PREPARATION
5 MINS

COOKING
10 MINS

SERVINGS
2

INGREDIENTS

- 6 slices of beef roast

- ½ tsp garlic powder

- 1/3 tsp dried thyme

- ¼ tsp dried rosemary

- 2 tbsp butter, unsalted

- Seasoning:

- 1/3 tsp salt

- 1/4 tsp ground black pepper

NUTRIRION

- Calories: 140

- Fats: 12.7 g

- Protein: 5.5 g

- Net Carbohydrates: 0.1 g

- Fiber: 0.2 g

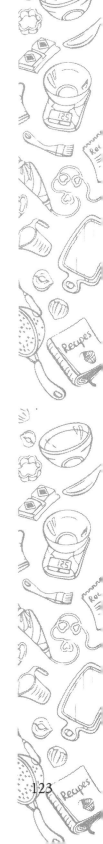

DIRECTIONS

1. Prepare the spice mix and for this, take a small bowl, place garlic powder, thyme, rosemary, salt, and black pepper and then stir until mixed.

2. Sprinkle spice mix on the beef roast.

3. Take a medium skillet pan, place it over medium heat, add butter and when it melts, add beef roast and then cook for 5 to 8 minutes until golden brown and cooked.

4. Serve.

Sprouts Stir-fry with Kale, Broccoli, and Beef

PREPARATION
5 MINS

COOKING
8 MINS

SERVINGS
2

INGREDIENTS

- 3 slices of beef roast, chopped
- 2 oz Brussels sprouts, halved
- 4 oz broccoli florets
- 3 oz kale
- 1 ½ tbsp butter, unsalted

- 1/8 tsp red pepper flakes
- Seasoning:
- ¼ tsp garlic powder
- ¼ tsp salt
- 1/8 tsp ground black pepper

NUTRIRION

- Calories: 140
- Fats: 12.7 g
- Protein: 5.5 g

- Net Carbohydrates: 0.1 g
- Fiber: 0.2 g

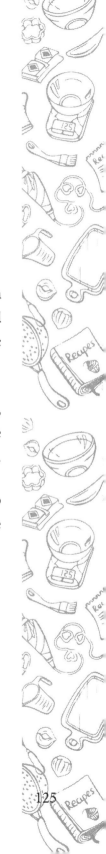

DIRECTIONS

1. Take a medium skillet pan, place it over medium heat, add ¾ tbsp butter and when it melts, add broccoli florets and sprouts, sprinkle with garlic powder, and cook for 2 minutes.

2. Season vegetables with salt and red pepper flakes, add chopped beef, stir until mixed and continue cooking for 3 minutes until browned on one side.

3. Then add kale along with remaining butter, flip the vegetables and cook for 2 minutes until kale leaves wilts.

4. Serve.

BEEF AND VEGETABLE SKILLET

PREPARATION
5 MINS

COOKING
15 MINS

SERVINGS
2

INGREDIENTS

- 3 oz spinach, chopped

- ½ pound ground beef

- 2 slices of bacon, diced

- 2 oz chopped asparagus

- Seasoning:

- 3 tbsp coconut oil

- 2 tsp dried thyme

- 2/3 tsp salt

- ½ tsp ground black pepper

NUTRIRION

- Calories 332.5

- Fats 26 g;

- Protein 23.5 g;

- Carbohydrates 1.5 g

- Fiber 1 g

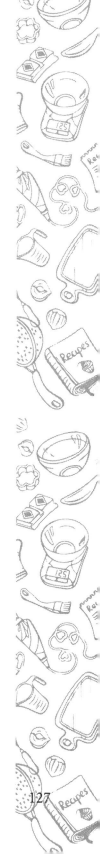

DIRECTIONS

1. Take a skillet pan, place it over medium heat, add oil and when hot, add beef and bacon and cook for 5 to 7 minutes until slightly browned.

2. Then add asparagus and spinach, sprinkle with thyme, stir well and cook for 7 to 10 minutes until thoroughly cooked.

3. Season skillet with salt and black pepper and serve.

Beef, Pepper and Green Beans Stir-fry

PREPARATION
5 MINS

COOKING
18 MINS

SERVINGS
2

INGREDIENTS

- 6 oz ground beef

- 2 oz chopped green bell pepper

- 4 oz green beans

- 3 tbsp grated cheddar cheese

- Seasoning:

- ½ tsp salt

- ¼ tsp ground black pepper

- ¼ tsp paprika

NUTRIRION

- Calories: 282.5

- Fats: 17.6 g

- Protein: 26.1 g

- Net Carbohydrates: 2.9 g

DIRECTIONS

1. Take a skillet pan, place it over medium heat, add ground beef and cook for 4 minutes until slightly browned.

2. Then add bell pepper and green beans, season with salt, paprika, and black pepper, stir well and continue cooking for 7 to 10 minutes until beef and vegetables have cooked through.

3. Sprinkle cheddar cheese on top, then transfer pan under the broiler and cook for 2 minutes until cheese has melted and the top is golden brown. And serve

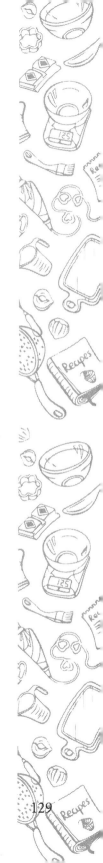

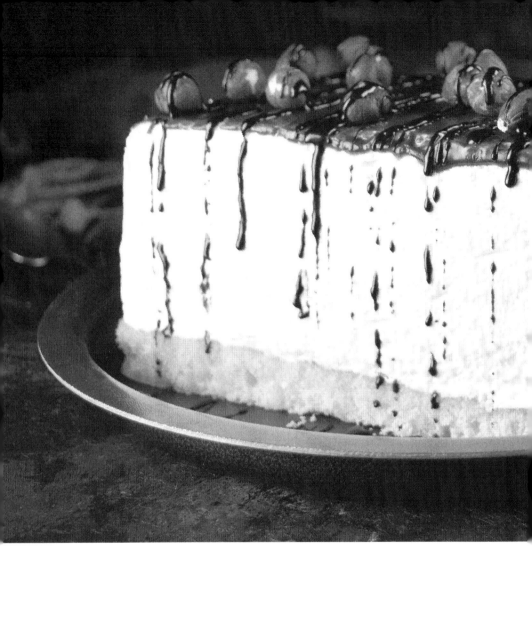

CHAPTER 09

DESSERT

Keto Cheesecakes

PREPARATION
25 MINS

SERVINGS
6

INGREDIENTS

- **For the cheesecakes:**

- 2 tablespoons butter

- 1 tablespoon caramel syrup; sugar-free

- 3 tablespoons coffee

- 8 ounces cream cheese

- 1/3 cup swerve sweetener

- 3 eggs

- **For the frosting:**

- 8 ounces mascarpone cheese; soft

- 3 tablespoons caramel syrup; sugar-free

- 2 tablespoons swerve

- 3 tablespoons butter

NUTRIRION

- Calories: 478.2

- Total Fat: 47.8 g

- Cholesterol: 140.4 mg

- Sodium : 270.7 mg

- Potassium: 233.7 mg

- Total Carbohydrate: 9.4 g

- Protein: 9.2 g

DIRECTIONS

1. In your blender, mix cream cheese with eggs, 2 tablespoons butter, coffee, 1 tablespoon caramel syrup, and 1/3 cup swerve. Pulse very well.

2. Spoon this into a cupcakes pan, introduce in the oven at 350 degrees F and bake for 15 minutes

3. Leave aside to cool down and then keep in the freezer for 3 hours

4. Meanwhile, in a bowl, mix 3 tablespoons butter with 3 tablespoons caramel syrup, 2 tablespoons swerve, and mascarpone cheese and blend well.

5. Spoon this over cheesecakes and serve them.

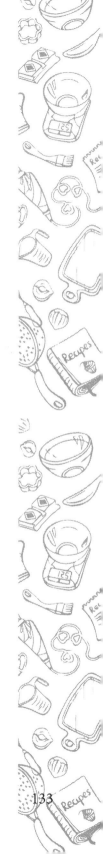

KETO BROWNIES

PREPARATION
30 MINS

SERVINGS
12

INGREDIENTS

- 6 ounces coconut oil; melted

- 4 ounces cream cheese

- 5 tablespoons swerve sweetener

- 6 eggs

- 2 teaspoons vanilla

- 3 ounces of cocoa powder

- 1/2 teaspoon baking powder

NUTRIRION

- Calories: 183.7

- Total Fat: 16.6 g

- Cholesterol: 20.7 mg

- Sodium : 36.3 mg

- Potassium: 21.6 mg

- Total Carbohydrate: 4.9 g

- Protein: 1.4 g

DIRECTIONS

1. In a blender, mix eggs with coconut oil, cocoa powder, baking powder, vanilla, cream cheese, and swerve. Stir using a mixer.

2. Pour this into a lined baking dish, introduce in the oven at 350 degrees F and bake for 20 minutes

3. Slice into rectangle pieces when it gets cold and serve

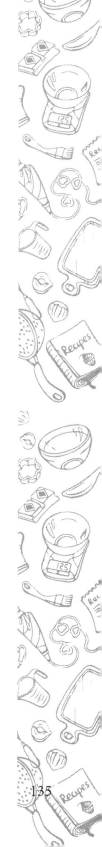

Raspberry and Coconut

PREPARATION
15 MINS

SERVINGS
12

INGREDIENTS

- 1/4 cup swerve sweetener

- 1/2 cup coconut oil

- 1/2 cup raspberries; dried

- 1/2 cup coconut; shredded

- 1/2 cup coconut butter

NUTRIRION

- Carbohydrates: 45g

- Sugar: 30g

- Fat: 42g

- Protein: 8g

- Cholesterol: 0mg

DIRECTIONS

1. In your food processor, blend dried berries very well.

2. Heat a pan with the butter over medium heat.

3. Add oil, coconut and swerve; stir and cook for 5 minutes

4. Pour half of this into a lined baking pan and spread well.

5. Add raspberry powder and also spread.

6. Top with the rest of the butter mix, spread and keep in the fridge for a while

7. Cut into pieces and serve

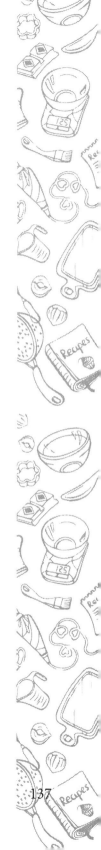

Chocolate Pudding Delight

PREPARATION
52 MINS

SERVINGS
2

INGREDIENTS

- 1/2 teaspoon stevia powder

- 2 tablespoons cocoa powder

- 2 tablespoons water

- 1 tablespoon gelatin

- 1 cup of coconut milk

- 2 tablespoons maple syrup

NUTRIRION

- Calories: 221.2

- Total Fat: 13.6 g

- Cholesterol: 9.8 mg

- Sodium : 250.3 mg

- Potassium: 86.7 mg

- Total Carbohydrate: 22.7 g

- Protein: 3.4 g

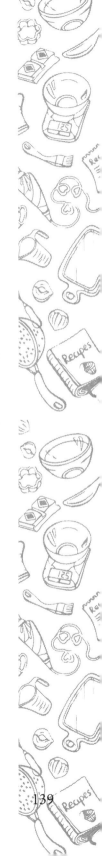

DIRECTIONS

1. Heat a pan with the coconut milk over medium heat; add stevia and cocoa powder and mix well.

2. In a bowl, mix gelatin with water; stir well and add to the pan.

3. Stir well, add maple syrup, whisk again, divide into ramekins and keep in the fridge for 45 minutes Serve cold.

Peanut Butter Fudge

PREPARATION
132 MINS

SERVINGS
12

INGREDIENTS

- 1 cup peanut butter; unsweetened

- 1 cup of coconut oil

- 1/4 cup almond milk

- 2 teaspoons vanilla stevia

- A pinch of salt

- For the topping:

- 2 tablespoons swerve sweetener

- 1/4 cup cocoa powder

- 2 tablespoons melted coconut oil

NUTRIRION

- Calories: 85

- Fat: 4.7g

- Saturated Fat: 2.7g

- Protein: 0.5g

DIRECTIONS

1. In a heatproof bowl, mix peanut butter with 1 cup coconut oil; stir and heat up in your microwave until it melts

2. Add a pinch of salt, almond milk, and stevia; stir well everything and pour into a lined loaf pan.

3. Keep in the fridge for 2 hours and then slice it.

4. In a bowl, mix 2 tablespoons melted coconut with cocoa powder and swerve and stir very well.

5. Drizzle the sauce over your peanut butter fudge and serve

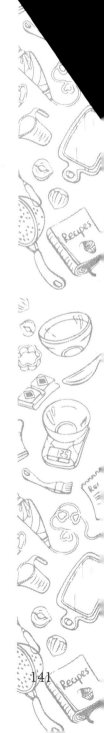

STREUSEL EGG LOAF

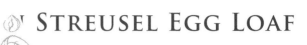

COOKING
15 MINS

SERVINGS
2

INGREDIENTS

- 2 tbsp almond flour

- 1 tbsp butter, softened

- ½ tbsp grated butter, chilled

- 1 egg

- 1-ounce cream cheese

- Others:

- ½ tsp cinnamon, divided

- 1 tbsp erythritol sweetener, divided

- ¼ tsp vanilla extract, unsweetened

NUTRIRION

- Calories: 152

- Fats: 14.8 g

- Protein: 4.1 g

- Net Carbohydrates: 1.3 g

- Fiber: 0.9 g

DIRECTIONS

1. Turn on the oven, then set it to 350 degrees F and let it preheat.

2. Meanwhile, crack the egg in a small bowl, add cream cheese, softened butter, ¼ tsp cinnamon, ½ tbsp sweetener, and vanilla and whisk until well combined.

3. Divide the egg batter between two silicone muffins and then bake for 7 minutes.

4. Meanwhile, prepare the streusel and for this, place flour in a small bowl, add remaining ingredients and stir until well mixed.

5. When egg loaves have baked, sprinkle streusel on top and then continue baking for 7 minutes.

6. When done, remove loaves from the cups, let them cool for 5 minutes and then serve and enjoy!

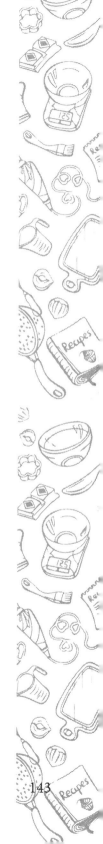

Snickerdoodle Muffins

PREPARATION
10 MINS

COOKING
12 MINS

SERVINGS
2

INGREDIENTS

- 6 2/3 tbsp coconut flour

- ½ of egg

- 1 tbsp butter, unsalted, melted

- 1 1/3 tbsp whipping cream

- 1 tbsp almond milk, unsweetened

- Others:

- 1 1/3 tbsp erythritol sweetener and more for topping

- ¼ tsp baking powder

- ¼ tsp ground cinnamon and more for topping

- ¼ tsp vanilla extract, unsweetened

NUTRIRION

- Calories: 241

- Fats: 21 g

- Protein: 7 g

- Net Carbohydrates: 3 g

- Fiber: 3 g

DIRECTIONS

1. Turn on the oven, then set it to 350 degrees F and let it preheat.

2. Meanwhile, take a medium bowl, place flour in it, add cinnamon and baking powder. Stir until combined.

3. Take a separate bowl, place the half egg in it, add butter, sour cream, milk, and vanilla and whisk until blended.

4. Whisk in flour mixture until a smooth batter is obtained, divide the batter evenly between two silicon muffin cups and then sprinkle cinnamon and sweetener on top.

5. Bake the muffins for 10 to 12 minutes until firm, and then the top has turned golden brown and then serve and enjoy!

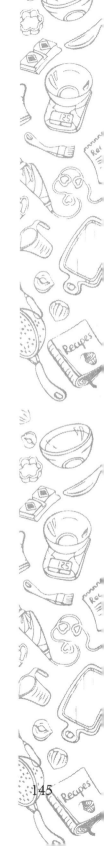

Yogurt and Strawberry Bowl

PREPARATION
5 MINS

COOKING
0 MINS

SERVINGS
2

INGREDIENTS

- 3 oz mixed berries
- 1 tbsp chopped almonds
- 1 tbsp chopped walnuts
- 4 oz yogurt

DIRECTIONS

1. Divide yogurt between two bowls, top with berries and then sprinkle with almonds and walnuts.

2. Serve and enjoy!

NUTRIRION

- Calories: 165
- Fats: 11.2 g
- Protein: 9.3 g
- Net Carbohydrates: 2.5 g
- Fiber: 1.8 g

Sweet Cinnamon M

PREPARATION
5 MINS

COOKING
2 MINS

SERVINGS
2

INGREDIENTS

- 4 tsp coconut flour

- 2 tsp cinnamon

- 2 tsp erythritol sweetener

- 1/16 tsp baking soda

- 2 eggs

DIRECTIONS

1. Take a medium bowl, place all the ingredients in it, and whisk until well combined.

2. Take two ramekins, grease them with oil, distribute the prepared batter in it and then microwave for 1 minute and 45 seconds until done.

3. When done, take out muffin from the ramekin, cut in half, and then serve and enjoy

NUTRIRION

- Calories: 101
- Fats: 6.5 g
- Protein: 7.6 g

- Net Carbohydrates: 0.5 g
- Fiber: 1.7 g

Nutty Muffins

PREPARATION
5 MINS

COOKING
5 MINS

SERVINGS
2

INGREDIENTS

- 4 tsp coconut flour
- 1/16 tsp baking soda
- 1 tsp erythritol sweetener
- 2 eggs
- 2 tsp almond butter, unsalted

NUTRIRION

- Calories: 131
- Fats: 8.6 g
- Protein: 8.4 g
- Net Carbohydrates: 2.3 g
- Fiber: 2.2 g

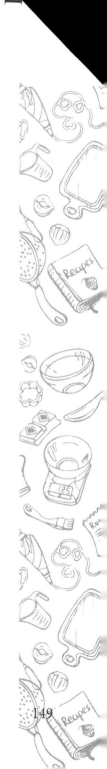

DIRECTIONS

1. Take a medium bowl, place all the ingredients in it, and whisk until well combined.

2. Take two ramekins, grease them with oil, distribute the prepared batter in it and then microwave for 1 minute and 45 seconds until done.

3. When done, take out muffin from the ramekin, cut in half, and then serve and enjoy!

PUMPKIN AND CREAM CHEESE CUP

PREPARATION
10 MINS

COOKING
12 MINS

SERVINGS
2

INGREDIENTS

- 4 tbsp almond flour

- 1 1/3 tbsp coconut flour

- 2 tbsp pumpkin puree

- 2 2/3 tbsp cream cheese, softened

- ½ of egg

- 2/3 tbsp butter, unsalted

- ¼ tsp pumpkin spice

- 2/3 tsp baking powder

- 2 tbsp erythritol sweetener

NUTRIRION

- Calories: 261

- Fats: 23 g

- Protein: 7 g

- Net Carbohydrates: 2 g

- Fiber: 4 g

DIRECTIONS

1. Turn on the oven, then set it to 350 degrees F and let it preheat.

2. Take a medium bowl, place butter and 1 ½ tbsp sweetener in it, and then beat until fluffy.

3. Beat in egg and then beat in pumpkin puree until well combined.

4. Take a medium bowl, place flours in it, stir in pumpkin spice, baking powder until mixed, stir this mixture into the butter mixture and then distribute it into two silicone muffin cups.

5. Take a medium bowl, place cream cheese in it, and stir in remaining sweetener until well combined.

6. Divide the cream cheese mixture into the silicone muffin cups, swirl the batter and cream cheese mixture by using a toothpick and then bake for 10 to 12 minutes until muffins have turned firm.

7. Serve and enjoy!

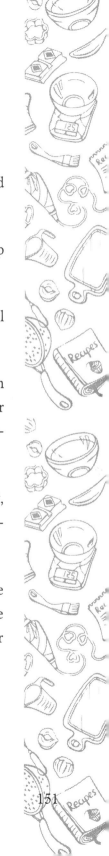

Berries in Yogurt Cream

PREPARATION
65 MINS

COOKING
0 MINS

SERVINGS
2

INGREDIENTS

- 1-ounce blackberries

- 1-ounce raspberry

- 2 tbsp erythritol sweetener

- 4 oz yogurt

- 4 oz whipping cream

NUTRIRION

- Calories: 245

- Fats: 22 g

- Protein: 4.2 g

- Net Carbohydrates: 5 g

- Fiber: 1.7

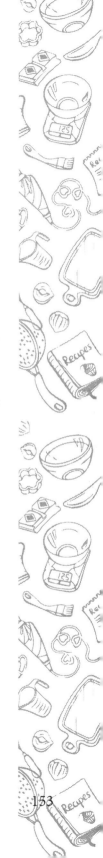

DIRECTIONS

1. Take a medium bowl, place yogurt in it, and then whisk in cream.

2. Sprinkle sweetener over yogurt mixture, don't stir, cover the bowl with a lid, and then refrigerate for 1 hour.

3. When ready to serve, stir the yogurt mixture, divide it evenly between two bowls, top with berries, and then serve and enjoy!

PUMPKIN PIE MUG CAKE

PREPARATION
5 MINS

COOKING
2 MINS

SERVINGS
2

INGREDIENTS

- 2 tbsp coconut flour

- 1 tsp sour cream

- 2 tbsp whipping cream

- 2 eggs

- ¼ cup pumpkin puree

- Others:

- 2 tbsp erythritol sweetener

- 1/3 tsp cinnamon

- ¼ tsp baking soda

NUTRIRION

- Calories: 245

- Fats: 22 g

- Protein: 4.2 g

- Net Carbohydrates: 5 g

- Fiber: 1.7

DIRECTIONS

1. Take a small bowl, place cream in it, and then beat in sweetener until well combined.

2. Cover the bowl, let it chill in the refrigerator for 30 minutes, then beat in eggs and pumpkin puree and stir in remaining ingredients until incorporated and smooth.

3. Divide the batter between two coffee mugs greased with oil and then microwave for 2 minutes until thoroughly cooked.

4. Serve and enjoy!

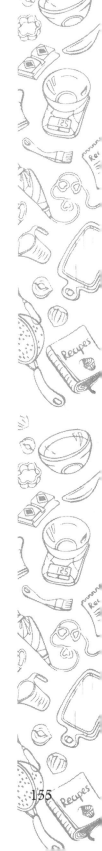

CHOCOLATE AND STRAWBERRY CREPE

PREPARATION
5 MINS

COOKING
5 MINS

SERVINGS
2

INGREDIENTS

- 1 1/3 tbsp coconut flour

- 1 tsp of cocoa powder

- ¼ tsp flaxseed

- 1 egg

- 2 ¾ tbsp coconut milk,

unsweetened

- 2 tsp avocado oil

- 1/8 tsp baking powder

- 2 oz strawberry, sliced

NUTRIRION

- Calories 120

- Fats 8.5 g

- Protein 4.4 g

- Carbohydrates 2.8 g

- Fiber 2.7 g

DIRECTIONS

1. Take a medium bowl, place flour in it, and then stir in cocoa powder, baking powder, and flaxseed in it until mixed.

2. Add egg and milk and then whisk until smooth.

3. Take a medium skillet pan, place it over medium heat, add 1 tsp oil and when hot, pour in half of the batter, spread it evenly, and then cook for 1 minute per side until firm.

4. Transfer crepe to a plate, add remaining oil, and cook another crepe by using the remaining batter.

5. When done, fill crepes with strawberries, fold them and then serve and enjoy

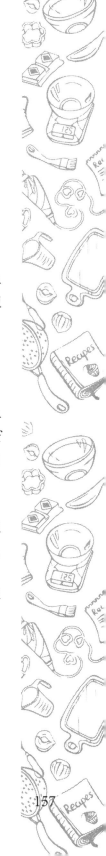

BLACKBERRY AND COCONUT FLOUR CUPCAKE

PREPARATION
5 MINS

COOKING
15 MINS

SERVINGS
2

INGREDIENTS

- 3 ¼ tbsp coconut flour

- 1/3 cup whipping cream

- 1 tbsp cream cheese

- 1 ½ egg

- 1-ounce blackberry

- 2 2/3 tbsp butter, unsalted,

chopped

- 5 1/3 tbsp erythritol sweetener

- 2/3 tsp baking powder

- 1/3 tsp vanilla extract, unsweetened

NUTRIRION

- Calorie: 420

- Fats: 38.2 g

- Protein: 9.4 g

- Net Carbohydrates: 5.7 g

- Fiber: 4.8 g

DIRECTIONS

1. Take a small bowl, place butter in it, add cream and them microwave for 30 to 60 seconds until it melts, stirring every 20 seconds.

2. Then add cream cheese, cream, vanilla, and erythritol, whisk until smooth, whisk in coconut flour and baking powder until incorporated and then fold in berries.

3. Distribute the mixture evenly between four muffin cups, then bake for 12 to 15 minutes until firm.

4. Serve and enjoy!

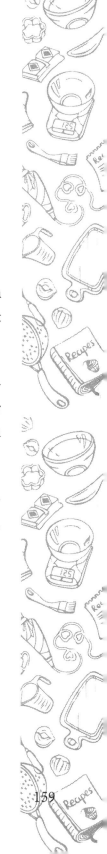

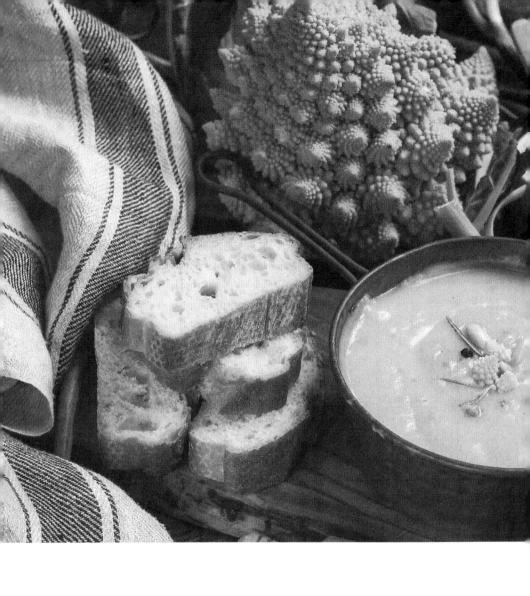

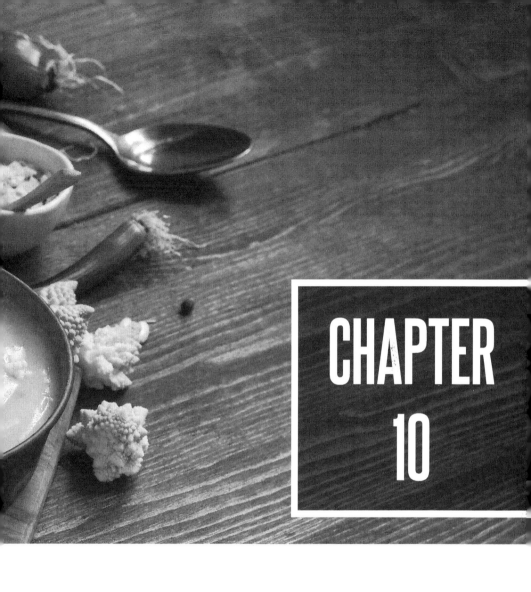

CHAPTER 10

SOUP

Coconut Soup

PREPARATION
12 MINS

COOKING
35 MINS

SERVINGS
4

INGREDIENTS

- 2 cloves garlic

- 1 medium white onion

- 1 tbsp butter

- 2 cups of water

- 2 cups vegetable stock

- 1 cup heavy cream

- Salt and ground black pepper to taste

- ½ tsp paprika

- 1½ cups broccoli, divided into florets

- 1 cup cheddar cheese

NUTRIRION

- Calories: 348

- Carbohydrates: 6.8g

- Fat: 33.8g

- Protein: 10.9g

DIRECTIONS

1. Peel and mince garlic. Peel and chop the onion.

2. Preheat pot on medium heat, add butter and melt it.

3. Add garlic and onion and sauté for 5 minutes, stirring occasionally.

4. Pour in water, vegetable stock, heavy cream, and add pepper, salt, and paprika.

5. Stir and bring to boil.

6. Add broccoli and simmer for 25 minutes.

7. After that, transfer soup mixture to a food processor and blend well.

8. Grate cheddar cheese and add to a food processor, blend again.

9. Serve soup hot.

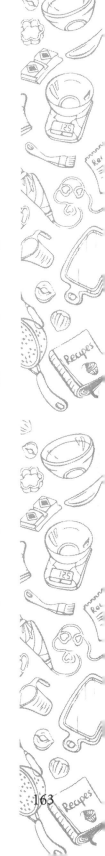

Broccoli Soup

PREPARATION
12 MINS

COOKING
35 MINS

SERVINGS
4

INGREDIENTS

- 2 cloves garlic

- 1 medium white onion

- 1 tbsp butter

- 2 cups of water

- 2 cups vegetable stock

- 1 cup heavy cream

- Salt and ground black pepper to taste

- ½ tsp paprika

- 1½ cups broccoli, divided into florets

- 1 cup cheddar cheese

NUTRIRION

- Calories: 348

- Carbohydrates: 6.8g

- Fat: 33.8g

- Protein: 10.9g

DIRECTIONS

1. Peel and mince garlic. Peel and chop the onion.

2. Preheat pot on medium heat, add butter and melt it.

3. Add garlic and onion and sauté for 5 minutes, stirring occasionally.

4. Pour in water, vegetable stock, heavy cream, and add pepper, salt, and paprika.

5. Stir and bring to boil.

6. Add broccoli and simmer for 25 minutes.

7. After that, transfer soup mixture to a food processor and blend well.

8. Grate cheddar cheese and add to a food processor, blend again.

9. Serve soup hot.

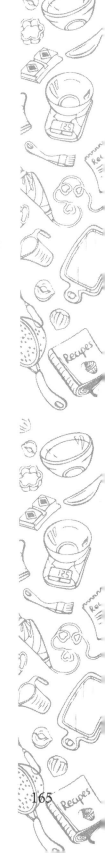

Simple Tomato Soup

PREPARATION
15 MINS

COOKING
10 MINS

SERVINGS
6

INGREDIENTS

- 4 cups canned tomato soup

- 2 tbsp apple cider vinegar

- 1 tsp dried oregano

- 4 tbsp butter

- 2 tsp turmeric

- 2 oz red hot sauce

- Salt and ground black pepper

to taste

- 4 tbsp olive oil

- 8 bacon strips, cooked and crumbled

- 4 oz fresh basil leaves, chopped

- 4 oz green onions, chopped

NUTRIRION

- Calories: 397

- Carbohydrates: 9.8g

- Fat: 33.8

- Protein: 11.7g

DIRECTIONS

1. Pour tomato soup in the pot and preheat on medium heat. Bring to boil.

2. Add vinegar, oregano, butter, turmeric, hot sauce, salt, black pepper, and olive oil. Stir well.

3. Simmer the soup for 5 minutes.

4. Serve soup topped with crumbled bacon, green onion, and basil.

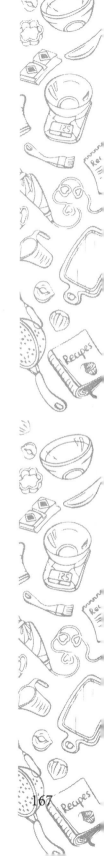

GREEN SOUP

PREPARATION
12 MINS

COOKING
15 MINS

SERVINGS
6

INGREDIENTS

- 2 cloves garlic

- 1 white onion

- 1 cauliflower head

- 2 oz butter

- 1 bay leaf, crushed

- 1 cup spinach leaves

- ½ cup watercress

- 4 cups vegetable stock

- Salt and ground black pepper to taste

- 1 cup of coconut milk

- ½ cup parsley, for serving

NUTRIRION

- Calories: 227

- Carbohydrates: 4.89g

- Fat: 35.1

- Protein: 6.97g

DIRECTIONS

1. Peel and mince garlic. Peel and dice onion.

2. Divide cauliflower into florets.

3. Preheat pot on medium-high heat, add butter and melt it.

4. Add onion and garlic, stir, and sauté for 4 minutes.

5. Add cauliflower and bay leaf, stir and cook for 5 minutes.

6. Add spinach and watercress, stir and cook for another 3 minutes.

7. Pour in vegetable stock—season with salt and black pepper. Stir and bring to boil.

8. Pour in coconut milk and stir well. Take off heat.

9. Use an immersion blender to blend well.

10. Top with parsley and serve hot.

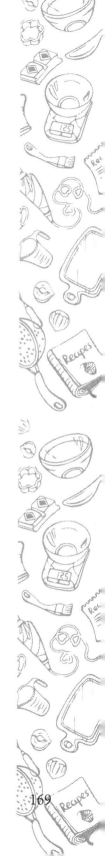

Sausage and Peppers Soup

PREPARATION
15 MINS

COOKING
75 MINS

SERVINGS
6

INGREDIENTS

- 1 tbsp avocado oil

- 2 lbs pork sausage meat

- Salt and ground black pepper to taste

- 1 green bell pepper, seeded and chopped

- 5 oz canned jalapeños, chopped

- 5 oz canned tomatoes, chopped

- 1¼ cup spinach

- 4 cups beef stock

- 1 tsp Italian seasoning

- 1 tbsp cumin

- 1 tsp onion powder

- 1 tsp garlic powder

- 1 tbsp chili powder

NUTRIRION

- Calories: 227

- Carbohydrates: 4.89g

- Fat: 35.1

- Protein: 6.97g

DIRECTIONS

1. Preheat pot with avocado oil on medium heat.

2. Put sausage meat in pot and brown for 3 minutes on all sides.

3. Add salt, black pepper, and green bell pepper and continue to cook for 3 minutes.

4. Add jalapeños and tomatoes, stir well and cook for 2 minutes more.

5. Toss spinach and stir again close lid and cook for 7 minutes.

6. Pour in beef stock, Italian seasoning, cumin, onion powder, chili powder, garlic powder, salt, and black pepper, stir well. Close lid again. Cook for 30 minutes.

7. When time is up, uncover the pot and simmer for 15 minutes more.

8. Serve hot.

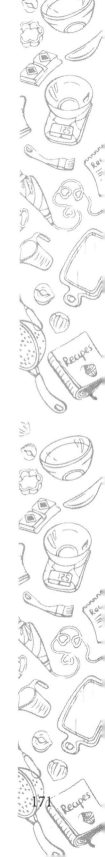

Avocado Soup

PREPARATION
12 MINS

COOKING
15 MINS

SERVINGS
4

INGREDIENTS

- 2 tbsp butter

- 2 scallions, chopped

- 3 cups chicken stock

- 2 avocados, pitted, peeled, and chopped

- Salt and ground black pepper to taste

- ⅔ cup heavy cream

NUTRIRION

- Calories: 329

- Carbohydrates: 5.9g

- Fat: 22.9g

- Protein: 5.8g

DIRECTIONS

1. Preheat pot on medium heat, add butter and melt it.

2. Toss scallions, stir and sauté for 2 minutes.

3. Pour in 2 ½ cups stock and bring to simmer—Cook for 3 minutes.

4. Meanwhile, peel and chop avocados.

5. Place avocado, ½ cup of stock, cream, salt, and pepper in a blender and blend well.

6. Add avocado mixture to the pot and mix well—Cook for 2 minutes.

7. Sprinkle with more salt and pepper, stir.

8. Serve hot.

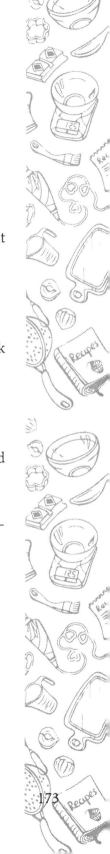

AVOCADO AND BACON SOUP

PREPARATION
15 MINS

COOKING
15 MINS

SERVINGS
6

INGREDIENTS

- 1-quart chicken stock

- 2 avocados, pitted

- ⅓ cup fresh cilantro, chopped

- 1 tsp garlic powder

- Salt and ground black pepper

to taste

- Juice of ½ lime

- ½ lb bacon, cooked and chopped

NUTRIRION

- Calories: 298

- Carbohydrates: 5.98g

- Fat: 22.8g

- Protein: 16.8g

DIRECTIONS

1. Pour chicken stock in a pot and bring to boil over medium-high heat.

2. Meanwhile, peel and chop the avocados.

3. Place avocados, cilantro, garlic powder, salt, black pepper, and lime juice in blender or food processor and blend well.

4. Add the avocado mixture in boiling stock and stir well.

5. Add bacon and season with salt and pepper to taste.

6. Stir and simmer for 3-4 minutes on medium heat.

7. Serve hot.

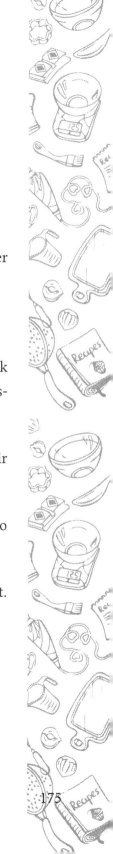

Roasted Bell Peppers Soup

PREPARATION
15 MINS

COOKING
20 MINS

SERVINGS
6

INGREDIENTS

- 1 medium white onion

- 2 cloves garlic

- 2 celery stalks

- 12 oz roasted bell peppers, seeded

- 2 tbsp olive oil

- Salt and ground black pepper

to taste

- 1-quart chicken stock

- 2/3 cup water

- ¼ cup Parmesan cheese, grated

- ⅔ cup heavy cream

NUTRIRION

- Calories: 180

- Carbohydrates: 3.9g

- Fat: 12.9g

- Protein: 5.9g

DIRECTIONS

1. Directions:

2. Peel and chop onion and garlic. Chop celery and bell pepper.

3. Preheat pot with oil on medium heat.

4. Put garlic, onion, celery, salt, and pepper in the pot, stir and sauté for 8 minutes.

5. Pour in chicken stock and water. Add bell peppers and stir.

6. Bring to boil, close lid, and simmer for 5 minutes. Reduce heat if needed.

7. When time is up, blend soup using an immersion blender.

8. Add cream and season with salt and pepper to taste. Take off heat.

9. Serve hot with grated cheese.

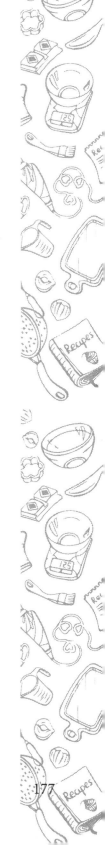

Spicy Bacon Soup

PREPARATION
15 MINS

COOKING
30 MINS

SERVINGS
6

INGREDIENTS

- 10 oz bacon, chopped

- Salt to taste

- 1 tbsp olive oil

- 2/3 cup cauliflower, divided into florets

- 4 oz green bell pepper, seeded and chopped

- 1 jalapeno pepper, seeded and chopped

- 4 cups chicken stock

- 2 tbsp full-fat cream

- 1 tsp ground black pepper

- 1 tsp chili pepper

NUTRIRION

- Calories: 301

- Carbohydrates: 3.9g

- Fat: 23g

- Protein: 19g

DIRECTIONS

1. In a bowl, combine bacon with salt.

2. Heat a pan over medium heat and cook bacon for 5 minutes, stirring constantly.

3. Remove bacon from pan and set aside.

4. Pour olive oil in a pan and add cauliflower, bell pepper, and jalapeno.

5. Cook veggies on high heat for 1 minute, stirring occasionally.

6. In a saucepan, mix bacon with vegetables. Pour in chicken stock. Stir.

7. Close lid and cook for 20-25 minutes.

8. Open the lid and add cream, stir.

9. Season with salt, black pepper, and chili pepper. Stir and cook for 5 minutes more.

10. Serve.

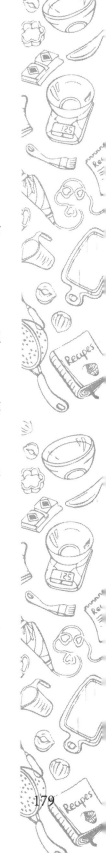

Italian Sausage Soup

PREPARATION
15 MINS

COOKING
35 MINS

SERVINGS
10

INGREDIENTS

- 1 tsp avocado oil

- 2 cloves garlic

- 1 medium white onion

- 1½ lbs hot pork sausage, chopped

- 8 cups chicken stock

- 1 lb radishes, chopped

- 10 oz spinach

- 1 cup heavy cream

- 6 bacon slices, chopped

- Salt and ground black pepper to taste

- A pinch of red pepper flakes

NUTRIRION

- Calories: 289

- Carbohydrates: 3.8g

- Fat: 21.8g

- Protein: 18.1g

DIRECTIONS

1. Preheat pot on medium-high heat and add oil.

2. Peel and chop garlic and onion.

3. Put garlic, onion, and sausage in the pot and stir.

4. Cook for few minutes until browned.

5. Pour in chicken stock; add radishes and spinach, stir.

6. Bring mixture to simmer and add cream, bacon, black pepper, salt, and red pepper flakes, stir well.

7. Simmer for 20 minutes.

8. Serve hot.

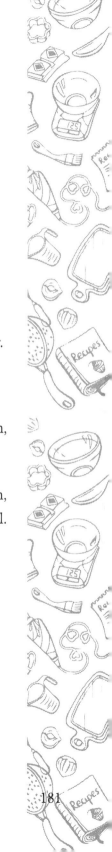

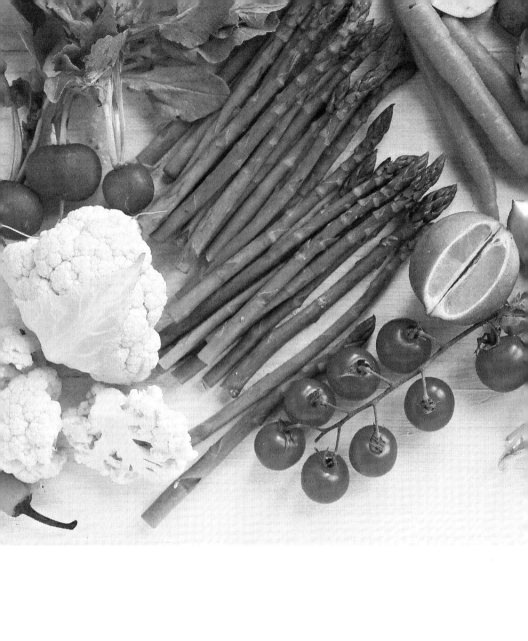

CHAPTER 11

VEGETABLES

Cabbage Hash Browns

PREPARATION
10 MINS

COOKING
12 MINS

SERVINGS
2

INGREDIENTS

- Ingredients
- 1 ½ cup shredded cabbage
- 2 slices of bacon
- 1/2 tsp garlic powder
- 1 egg

- Seasoning:
- 1 tbsp coconut oil
- ½ tsp salt
- 1/8 tsp ground black pepper

NUTRIRION

- Calories: 336
- Fats: 29.5 g
- Protein: 16 g

- Net Carbohydrates: 0.9 g
- Fiber: 0.8 g

DIRECTIONS

1. Crack the egg in a bowl, add garlic powder, black pepper, and salt, whisk well, then add cabbage, toss until well mixed and shape the mixture into four patties.

2. Take a large skillet pan, place it over medium heat, add oil and when hot, add patties in it and cook for 3 minutes per side until golden brown.

3. Transfer hash browns to a plate, then add bacon into the pan and cook for 5 minutes until crispy.

4. Serve hash browns with bacon.

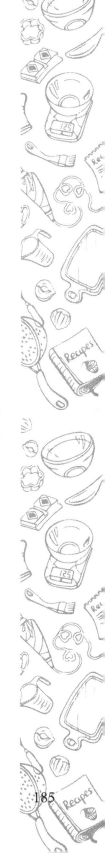

CAULIFLOWER HASH BROWNS

PREPARATION
10 MINS

COOKING
18 MINS

SERVINGS
2

INGREDIENTS

- ¾ cup grated cauliflower t

- 2 slices of bacon

- 1/2 tsp garlic powder

- 1 large egg white

- Seasoning:

- 1 tbsp coconut oil

- ½ tsp salt

- 1/8 tsp ground black pepper

NUTRIRION

- Calories: 347.8

- Fats: 31 g

- Protein: 15.6 g

- Net Carbohydrates: 1.2 g

- Fiber: 0.5 g

DIRECTIONS

1. Place grated cauliflower in a heatproof bowl, cover with plastic wrap, poke some holes in it with a fork and then microwave for 3 minutes until tender.

2. Let steamed cauliflower cool for 10 minutes, then wrap in a cheesecloth and squeeze well to drain moisture as much as possible.

3. Crack the egg in a bowl, add garlic powder, black pepper, and salt, whisk well, then add cauliflower and toss until well mixed and sticky mixture comes together.

4. Take a large skillet pan, place it over medium heat, add oil and when hot, drop cauliflower mixture on it, press lightly to form hash brown patties, and cook for 3 to 4 minutes per side until browned.

5. Transfer hash browns to a plate, then add bacon into the pan and cook for 5 minutes until crispy.

6. Serve hash browns with bacon.

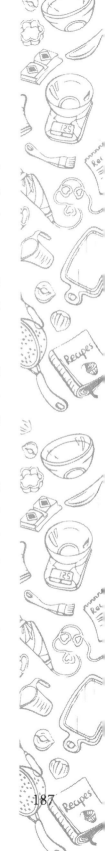

ASPARAGUS, WITH BACON AND EGGS

PREPARATION
5 MINS

COOKING
12 MINS

SERVINGS
2

INGREDIENTS

- 4 oz asparagus

- 2 slices of bacon, diced

- 1 egg

- Seasoning:

- ¼ tsp salt

- 1/8 tsp ground black pepper

NUTRIRION

- Calories: 179

- Fats: 15.3 g

- Protein: 9 g

- Net Carbohydrates: 0.7 g

- Fiber: 0.6 g

DIRECTIONS

1. Take a skillet pan, place it over medium heat, add bacon, and cook for 4 minutes until crispy.

2. Transfer cooked bacon to a plate, then add asparagus into the pan and cook for 5 minutes until tender-crisp.

3. Crack the egg over the cooked asparagus, season with salt and black pepper, then switch heat to medium-low level and cook for 2 minutes until the egg white has set.

4. Chop the cooked bacon slices, sprinkle over egg and asparagus and serve.

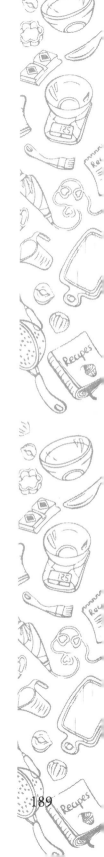

BELL PEPPER EGGS

PREPARATION
10 MINS

COOKING
4 MINS

SERVINGS
2

INGREDIENTS

- 1 green bell pepper

- 2 eggs

- Seasoning:

- 1 tsp coconut oil

- ¼ tsp salt

- ¼ tsp ground black pepper

NUTRIRION

- Calories: 110.5

- Fats: 8 g

- Protein: 7.2 g

- Net Carbohydrates: 1.7 g

- Fiber: 1.1 g

DIRECTIONS

1. Prepare pepper rings, and for this, cut out two slices from the pepper, about ¼-inch, and reserve remaining bell pepper for later use.

2. Take a skillet pan, place it over medium heat, grease it with oil, place pepper rings in it, and then crack an egg into each ring.

3. Season eggs with salt and black pepper, cook for 4 minutes, or until eggs have cooked to the desired level.

4. Transfer eggs to a plate and serve.

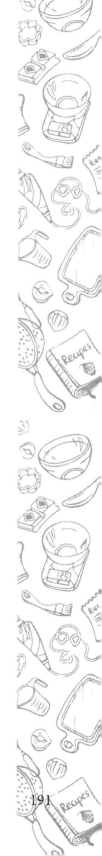

OMELET-STUFFED PEPPERS

PREPARATION
5 MINS

COOKING
20 MINS

SERVINGS
2

INGREDIENTS

- 1 large green bell pepper, halved, cored

- 2 eggs

- 2 slices of bacon, chopped, cooked

- 2 tbsp grated parmesan cheese

- Seasoning:

- 1/3 tsp salt

- ¼ tsp ground black pepper

NUTRIRION

- Calories: 428

- Fats: 35.2 g

- Protein: 23.5 g

- Net Carbohydrates: 2.8 g

- Fiber: 1.5

DIRECTIONS

1. Directions:

2. Turn on the oven, then set it to 400 degrees F, and let preheat.

3. Then take a baking dish, pour in 1 tbsp water, place bell pepper halved in it, cut-side up, and bake for 5 minutes.

4. Meanwhile, crack eggs in a bowl, add chopped bacon and cheese, season with salt and black pepper, and whisk until combined.

5. After 5 minutes of baking time, remove baking dish from the oven, evenly fill the peppers with egg mixture and continue baking for 15 to 20 minutes until eggs have set.

6. Serve.

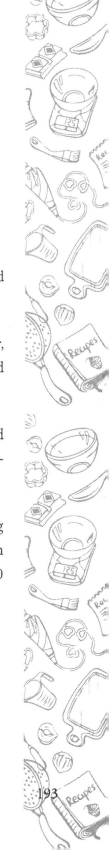

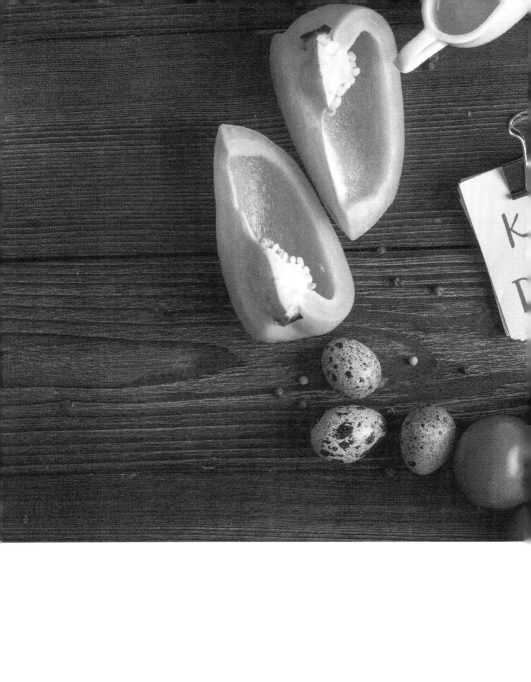

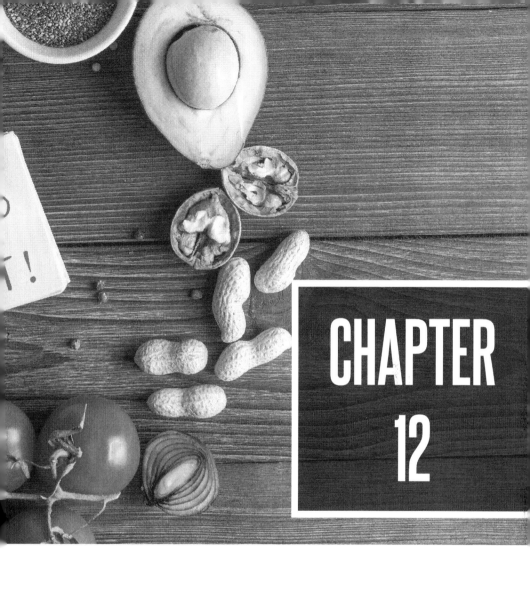

CHAPTER
12

CONCLUSION

Conclusion

The ketogenic diet is one that has many important aspects and information that you need to know as someone who wants to try this diet. It is important to remember the warning that we have given you at the beginning of the book that this is not a diet that is safe and that doctors don't recommend to try it, and if you are going to attempt it remember that you shouldn't do so for longer than six months and even then never without the constant supervision of a doctor or at the very least a doctor knowing that you're doing this and that you're following their guidelines and words to the letter so they can make sure you are safe.

The ketogenic diet is a diet that believes that by minimizing your carbs while maximizing the good fat in your system and making sure that you're getting the protein you need, you will be happier and healthier. In this guidebook, we give you the information to know what this diet is all about, as well as describing the different types and areas that this diet will offer. Most people assume that there is only one way to do this and while there is one thing that the additional options share, there are actually four different options you can choose from. Each one has its unique benefits, and you should know about each type to learn what would be best for your body, which is why we have described them in the book for you to have the best information possible when you begin this diet for yourself.

Another big thing about this diet is that many people don't understand the importance of exercise with this diet. The best way to become healthier is to do three things for yourself. Get the right amount of sleep, eat healthily, and make sure that you get the proper amount of exercise as well for your body to work at an optimum level. The exercises, such as the ones that we explained, are the best to go with your diet to make sure that you are getting the most out of it.

For women who are on the go and have a busy lifestyle, we have provided recipes for a thirty-day meal plan so that you can make food quickly and have a great meal for your lifestyle. They also have enough servings for you to have leftovers so that you don't have to worry about preparing more food in the morning. Instead, you can simply pack it up and take it with you wherever you go. This works out so much easier for so many people because they don't have to cook in the morning, and it saves a busy person a lot of time.

With all of this information at your fingertips, you will be able to enjoy this diet and use it to your advantage. Another benefit that we offer? We explain routines that you can do for yourself to make this diet last longer for you and to benefit your body better as a result. Routines are very important and can be a big help to your body but also your spirit and your mind. Good luck with your keto journey!